STUDENTS' GUIDE TO
HUMAN VIRUSES

STUDENTS' GUIDE TO
HUMAN VIRUSES

IGOR V. ZAITSEV

Library of Congress Control Number: 2014920824
ISBN: Hardcover   978-1-5035-1939-8
               Softcover   978-1-5035-1940-4
               eBook   978-1-5035-1941-1

The text provides concise and updated information on major human viruses, with emphasis on their structure and the diseases they may cause. The material is organized by using the viral classification approach as an alternative to the organ-system/disease approach. The text offers an overview of viral diseases for students and their instructors, clinicians, researches, and anyone in need of a thorough primer on the matter.

This book was printed in the United States of America.

Rev. date: 12/29/2014

To order additional copies of this book, contact:
Xlibris
1-888-795-4274
www.Xlibris.com
Orders@Xlibris.com
697661

TABLE OF CONTENTS

To Dr. Joseph A. Lieberman

FOREWORD

Students' Guide to Human Viruses offers comprehensive reviews of human viruses. The breadth and the format of this text make it particularly useful for college students and beginning microbiology instructors. Of note, it covers the material using the viral-classification approach as an alternative to the widely disseminated organ-system/disease approach referred to by many instructors as a "systemic approach." The latter became popular because a course on human anatomy and physiology is a prerequisite to Introductory Microbiology courses in most institutions of higher education. In that course, the human body is studied by the organ systems. Thus, it is usually assumed that students in microbiology courses would relate to the content more readily if diseases are covered by those systems. However, many pathogenic microorganisms, including viruses, affect not only one but at least a few systems. Since many viruses have diverse methods of replication and transmission as well as targeting multiple-cell types, assigning groups of viruses to a specific organ system may not be the most didactic alternative. Indeed, such a designation could be confusing, misleading, and difficult to comprehend since the organ-system approach places a secondary rather than a primary focus on the mechanism of viral infection. In order to provide a fresh teaching text for novice college microbiology instructors, the author offers an up-to-date compilation of human viral diseases, from DNA to RNA viruses. Each viral disease covered is first presented from the etiologic angle with useful tabular information and then expanded into the relevant aspects of its clinical signs and sequelae, incubation period, transmission, epidemiology, treatment, and prevention. Informative historical considerations are included as well.

This approach not only makes better sense theoretically but aids students in understanding and retaining the content in a more effective manner than that yielded by the systemic approach. It renders a powerful teaching tool for beginning instructors during their initial years of coping with the immense amount of information to be covered in preparation for their microbiology classes. At the same time, this text presents itself as a valuable resource for students of microbiology and infectious diseases as well as for anyone in need of a thorough primer on human viral diseases.

Alvaro Arjona, PhD
Director, Drug Development
GGO IP & Science Editorial
Thomson Reuters
Barcelona, Spain

CHAPTER I

General Characteristics Of Viruses

Outline

I. Viral Architecture

II. Viral Multiplication

    1. Attachment

    2. Penetration and Uncoating

    3. Phase of Synthesis: Replication

       • DNA Viruses

       • +ssRNA Viruses

       • −ssRNA Viruses

       • dsRNA Viruses

       • Retroviruses

    4. Maturation and Release

The virus is one of the great riddles of biology. We do not know whether it is alive or dead, because it seems to occupy a place midway between the inert chemical molecule and the living organism.

—Wendell Meredith Stanley, 1967

Viral Architecture

A virus is a subcellular parasitic entity composed of an infectious tightly folded and packed nucleic acid core within a protein shell called a capsid. The capsid is made up of structural units called capsomers, chains of polypeptides forming globular structures arranged in a precise fashion around the nucleic acid core. The mature viral particle as a unit is referred to as a virion. Virions have no organelles, but a number of them carry some enzymes inside their capsid. The capsid stabilizes the viral nucleic acid so that it survives in the outer environment and facilitates its entrance to susceptible cells. Some viruses are additionally surrounded by an envelope that they acquire during their release from the host cell. Those viruses are called enveloped viruses. The envelope is usually a piece of a cell membrane that viruses tear off from the cell while leaving it. Envelope viruses ordinarily do not lyse the host cell. The cell membrane could be either a plasma membrane or an endosomal membrane. Most of those viruses depend on the envelope for their infectivity. The most commonly enveloped viruses such as hepatitis B cause chronic infections. Some enveloped viruses are capable of causing acute infections with late sequelae—for example, the measles virus, which can cause a complication, subacute sclerosing panencephalitis, many years after the initial acute infection. They also can cause latent infections. A good example is a herpes simplex virus, whose nucleic acid is present in a host cell but does not actively produce the virus except under certain conditions. Viruses that do not possess an envelope are called naked viruses. Unlike enveloped viruses, naked viruses lyse the host cell in the release process. Consequently, they produce acute infections.

The viral binding proteins are scattered on the capsid and envelope surfaces. They help the virion to encounter just the right cell. Viruses are not considered as individual organisms but as infectious particles that do not have metabolism and are unable to reproduce independently from a parasitized host cell; they need a cellular machinery to multiply from a nucleic acid. Viruses have no energy, so they float around depending on a Brownian motion until they come in contact with a susceptible cell to start reproducing. The entry of viral nucleic acid into the host cell results in an infected cell that is then immune; it cannot be reinfected by the same or related viruses.

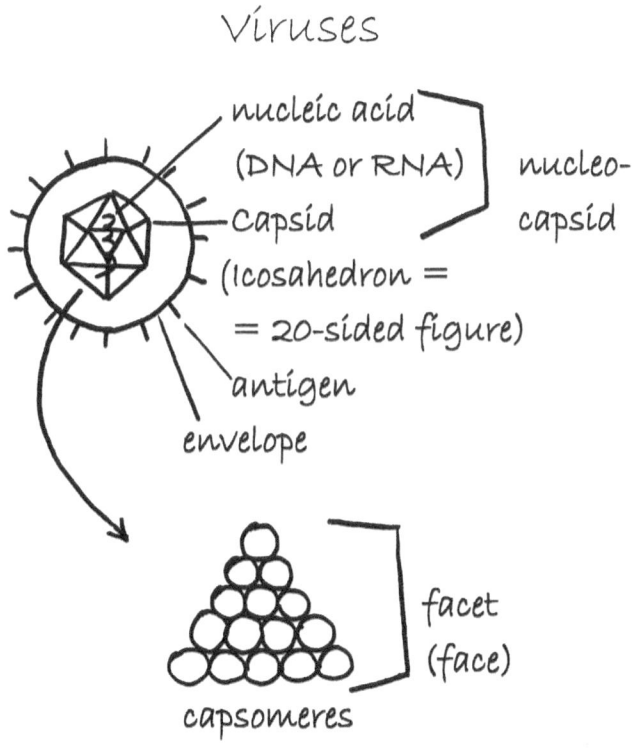

Figure 1.1. Viral architecture

Despite the fact that viruses are not of cellular organization, they are known to be highly complex structures. A highly purified preparation of virus is referred to as a virus crystal. There are three basic forms in the viral capsid structure:

- Icosahedral—a solid, many-sided geometric form in which the capsomers are arranged into twenty equilateral triangles (faces) and twelve apexes.
- Helical—a spiral, tubular structure bound up to make a compact mass. Only RNA viruses have helical symmetry. The capsomers are bound to RNA and coiled into a helical nucleoprotein capsid.
- Complex—variable structures in size and shape.

The genetic material (genome) in the capsid is either DNA or RNA, but never both. It could be organized with as little as 3 kb (1 kb = 1,000 nucleotides) genomes of viruses belonging to the family Hepadnaviridae or with as much as 380 kb double-stranded DNA (dsDNA) genomes of viruses belonging to the family Poxviridae. The strands of the nucleic acid are either single or paired. For example, the genome of human parvovirus B19, a virus that causes a form of childhood rash called erythema infectiosum or fifth disease, consists of single-stranded DNA (ssDNA). Hepatitis B virus is partially double-stranded, while an overwhelming majority of DNA viruses contain dsDNA. Human rotaviruses that cause a diarrheal disease contain double-stranded RNA (dsRNA); however, the vast majority of RNA viruses are single-stranded (ssRNA). It is important to keep in mind that the size of double-stranded genomes is expressed in base pairs (kbp) instead of just kb units.

The nucleic acid in the viral capsid is organized either in one continuous strand or in the separate segments. The HIV virus contains two segments of RNA in its capsid, influenza viruses eight segments of RNA, and rotaviruses eleven segments while the majority of others have nonsegmented genomes. The nucleic acid in the capsid could be either circular or linear. For instance, a virus causing genital warts contains covalently closed-circular dsDNA while most other viruses contain linear nucleic acids. All human papillomaviruses have circular dsDNA.

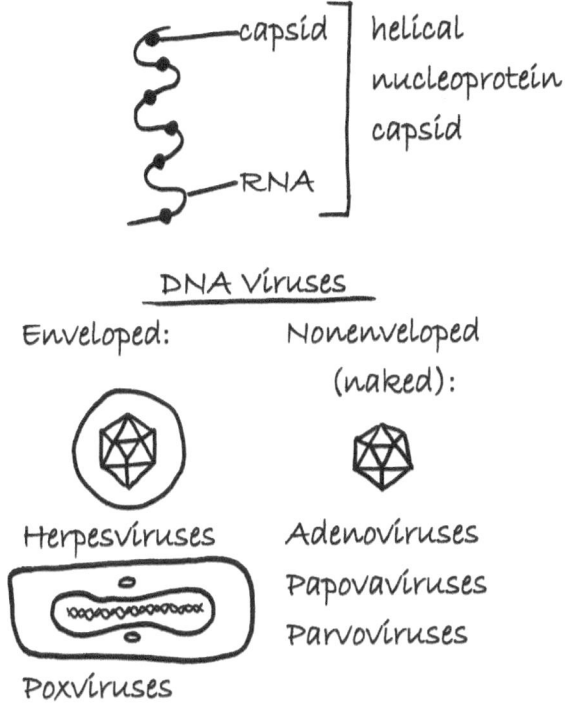

Figure 1.2. Capsids of DNA and RNA viruses

Viral Replication

Viral replication is a complex and very diverse process. Some steps may be overlapped; however, in general, it includes the following:

- Attachment, also known as adsorption
- Fusion and penetration
- Uncoating of the viral genome
- Transcription of early mRNA
- Transcription of early proteins
- Replication of viral nucleic acid
- Transcription of late mRNA
- Translation of late proteins
- Assembly of virions, also referred to as maturation
- Release of virions

Virions are attached to the specific cell receptors located on the outer surface of the cell membrane; cells that lack such receptors are not susceptible to viral infection. After an attachment, the virus penetrates the cell either by fusion of the viral envelope with the cell membrane or by initiating endocytosis in its target cell. The patterns of replication are very diverse and depend on the type of the genome the virus encompasses.

Attachment

An attachment or adsorption is the initial stage of the virus infection cycle of an animal. The surface of susceptible cells displays a protein or carbohydrate receptor that the virus uses as a binding side during their collision with the cell. Even though the viral surfaces are studded with attachment proteins, firm attachment will occur only if there is a certain affinity between the cell surface and the virion.

$$Replication$$

DNA viruses

$$DNA \rightarrow mRNA \rightarrow proteins$$

+RNA viruses

$$+RNA \rightarrow proteins$$

-RNA viruses

$$- RNA \rightarrow +RNA \rightarrow proteins$$

Retroviruses

$$RNA \rightarrow DNA \rightarrow mRNA \rightarrow$$
$$\rightarrow proteins$$

Figure 1.3. Protein synthesis by DNA and RNA viruses

Ordinarily, the virus host's cell binding occurs in several steps. Some viruses, before penetrating the cell, bind first to the accessory receptors, which usually have a low affinity, the process achieved due to electrostatic component. Then the virus is transferred to a high-affinity receptor. If an accessory receptor is not required by a certain virus, the high-affinity receptor plays the role of a primary receptor. In both cases, binding to it is an essential stage for the virus's entry into the cell. The host cells that do not express such a high-affinity receptor cannot be infected by the virus. In some cases, totally unrelated viruses use identical host receptors. For example, both Coxsackie viruses (RNA viruses) and many adenoviruses (DNA viruses) use the same CAR (coxsackie and adenovirus receptor) protein on the host cell. A sialic acid receptor is a receptor for many unrelated viruses (influenza virus, coronavirus, reovirus, etc.) expressed on many different cells and in many different organisms, which allows the potential virus to have a very wide host range. It is also uncommon for the same viral families to use a variety of different receptors.

Besides the requirement for a high-affinity receptor, many viruses require a coreceptor in order to enter the cell. For instance, HIV first binds to the primary receptor (human CD4 receptor) expressed on the surface of helper CD4+ T cells then binds to the coreceptor in order to penetrate the cell. Without a coreceptor on the susceptible cells, HIV is unable to produce any infections. As a result, some people whose cells do not express these coreceptors on the surfaces of their lymphocytes cannot be infected by the HIV. All receptors and coreceptors are specific, and a particular virus may be able to infect only a single or a limited number of cell types. A majority of viruses can infect only a single species.

Fusion, Penetration, and Uncoating

The next step contributing to a successful infection is the introduction of the viral genome into the cytoplasm of the cell. Some viruses simply inject their nucleic acid inside the cell while others introduce their nucleocapsid or an activated core particle.

In some viruses, the protein that promotes entry is the same as the proteins that bind to the receptor, while in others, it may be different proteins.

Penetration of enveloped animal viruses into a host cell depends on the nature of its envelope. Groups of viruses that acquired their envelopes from plasma membranes first activate their fusion (F) proteins, then their envelopes fuse with the susceptible cells before introducing the nucleocapsid into the cell cytoplasm.

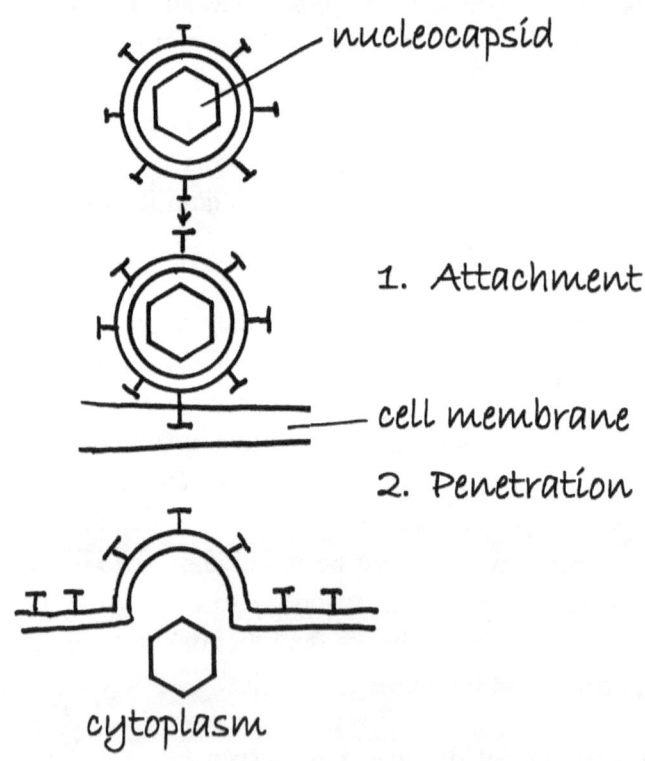

Figure 1.4. The attachment and penetration of viruses with a plasma membrane–acquired envelope

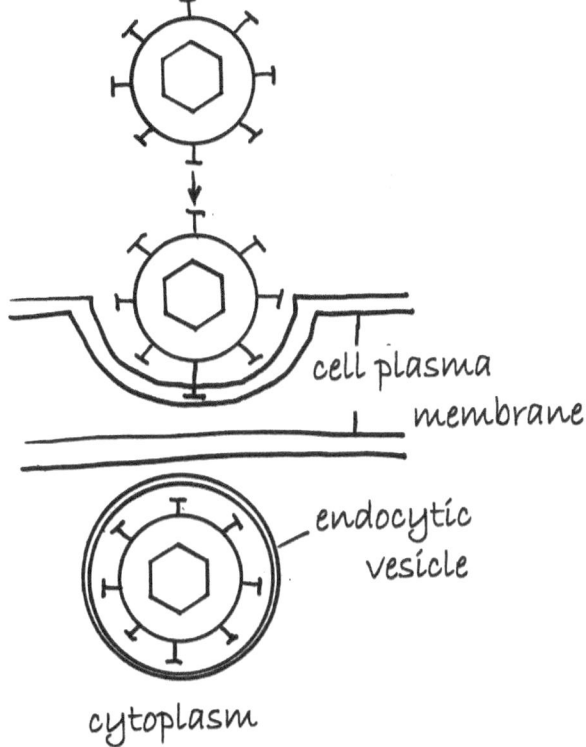

Figure 1.5. The attachment and penetration of viruses
with an endosome-acquired envelope

The viruses that possess endosomal envelopes infect cells
through an endocytic route. By binding to the plasma membrane
of the susceptible cell, they trigger the process of endocytosis and
become engulfed by the cell. They enter the cell in the clathrin-coated
endocytic vesicle. Clathrin is a protein that plays a major role in the
formation of such a vesicle. This clathrin-dependent endocytosis
accounts for the majority of uptakes from the plasma membrane. The
process of uncoating begins with the disappearance of a clathrin coat
while endosome becomes progressively acidified (~pH 5–6). The
acidic environment activates fusion protein and results in fusion of
the viral envelope with that of the endosome and, consequently, the
release of the nucleic acid into the cytosol.

Naked animal viruses, in contrast to their enveloped counterparts, cannot utilize membrane fusion to enter cells; instead they use penetration proteins, capsid proteins that mediate membrane penetration. Those proteins compromise the bilayer integrity, releasing the viral nucleic acids into the cytosol of the cell. A naked virus is also able to initiate receptor-mediated endocytosis, entering the cell in a vesicle. In general, this is the most common mechanism by which many hormones and toxins enter cells; the virion is engulfed and contained within an endocytic vesicle. However, only a few of the penetration processes of naked animal viruses are as yet only somewhat described and understood.

Phases of Synthesis: Replication

DNA Viruses

After penetration and uncoating, the DNA genome is transported to the nucleus via nuclear pores. In the nucleus, the first event in the replication of a DNA virus is the production of mRNA from the viral DNA. The expression of immediate early proteins allows initiation of viral genome duplication and early protein production, such as DNA polymerase, a protein that leads to the initiation of DNA replication and proteins that stimulate the cell to enter the S phase. Some polymers are required for further disassembly of subviral particles. In many viruses, DNA is transcribed by cellular RNA polymerase using the general mechanism of DNA replication. The process is similar even in single-stranded DNA viruses except that the single-stranded region must first be synthesized (+ strand → – strand → + strand).

Exception: Poxviruses are DNA viruses, but
they replicate in the cytoplasm.

In all eukaryotic cells, DNA replication is initiated by a specific RNA polymerase called primase, then RNA primers become extended (catalyzed) by DNA polymerase. The ribonucleotides in the primer are removed at the end of the replication by exonuclease. After that, DNA polymerase fills the gap, and ligase seals the nick. DNA polymerase can move only in a 5' → 3' direction and are never able to initiate a new DNA chain (it is the job of primase). Because of this, there is a problem of winding up the replication at the 5' end of a DNA molecule. For this reason, eukaryotic cells have a special region of repetitive nucleotides at the end of the genome called telomeres, which are disposable buffers blocking the ends of the DNA molecule so the cell will not lose any genetic information. With each cell division, they become shortened and have to be replenished by the telomerase reverse transcriptase. Instead of having telomerase, viruses and bacteria have a different solution to this biological problem. Bacteria and many DNA viruses have circular genomes. The linear genomes of some DNA viruses are cyclized before or during replication, and thus, they do not have to deal with the 5' end of the DNA molecule. However, adenoviruses have an instruction on how to build its own primer protein and, therefore, are capable of duplicating their linear genome.

In different viruses with circular DNA genome, there are also differences of the replication fork progression. In polyomaviruses, the replication fork proceeds in both directions with the production of two double-stranded circles, whereas in herpesviruses, the replication fork proceeds in one direction.

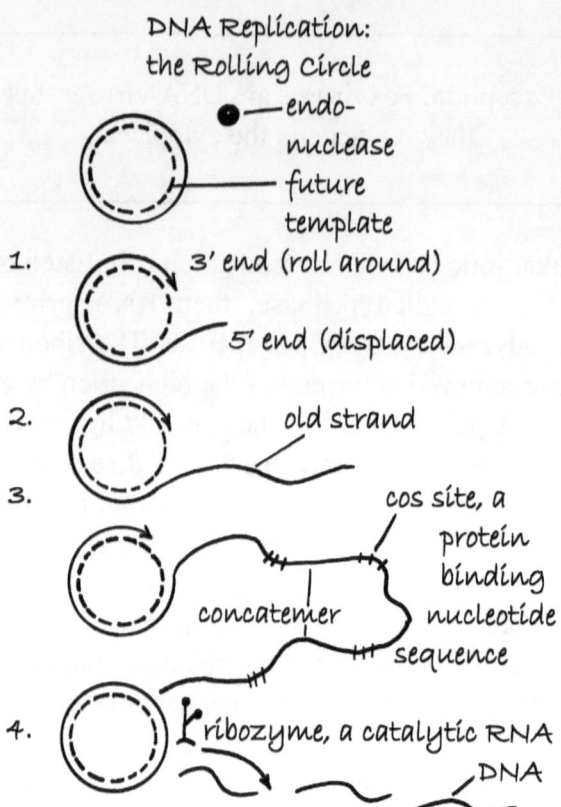

DNA Replication:
the Rolling Circle
● —endo-
      nuclease
      future
      template
1.   3' end (roll around)
      5' end (displaced)
2.   old strand
3.   cos site, a
        protein
        binding
concatemer   nucleotide
              sequence
4.   ribozyme, a catalytic RNA
                        DNA

Figure 1.6. The rolling circle of DNA replication:
(1) the DNA strand is nicked; (2) the 3' end is lengthened,
rolling around the circular template, and the 5' end is displaced;
(4) the formed strand of the multiple units is called a concatemer;
(5) the ribozyme, a catalytic RNA, cuts the concatemer.

Adenoviruses and herpesviruses have linear genomes, but their double-stranded DNA cyclize in preparation for replication. Their replication proceeds by what has been called a rolling circle, a mechanism that exclusively uses leading strand displacement synthesis, resulting in the production of concatemer—a long, continuous DNA molecule that contains multiple copies of the same DNA sequences linked in a series. In this mechanism, one strand is nicked by the endonuclease (an enzyme that cleaves the phosphodiester bond within a polynucleotide chain), exposing the 3' and 5' ends. The 3' end is extended by the DNA polymerase. The 5' end is displaced and forms a tail of single-stranded DNA that extends from the circle (concatemer).

The single-stranded tail is converted into a double-stranded tail by synthesis involving RNA primers as in the lagging strand of normal DNA replication. At one point, it becomes cleaved into separate DNA molecules by ribozymes (ribonucleic acid enzyme) or, as it sometimes called, catalytic RNA.

Positive Single-Stranded RNA Viruses

All eukaryotic positive single-stranded (+ssRNA) viruses replicate in the cytoplasm. The introduction of the naked +ssRNA into a susceptible cell results in a complete infection cycle because the cell's ribosomes recognize it as mRNA. The replication cycle begins by translating the RNA genome to produce the enzymes for RNA synthesis. A complementary negative-strand RNA is transcribed from the positive-strand RNA by viral RNA polymerase.

Negative Single-Stranded RNA Viruses

These viruses are a little more diverse and tend to have larger genomes encoding more genetic information than positive-stranded viruses. The nucleocapsid is helical, remaining intact during replication of the virus in the cell; its RNA is never released from it. Negative single-stranded RNA (–ssRNA) viruses must have their genome copied by an RNA polymerase to form positive-sense RNAs, which are translated into viral proteins required for synthesis. Among them are capsid proteins and RNA-dependent RNA polymerase, the enzyme that produces new negative-sense RNA molecules, and glycoproteins that are transported to the cell plasma membrane. Assembled nucleocapsids bud out through the areas of the plasma membrane where the viral glycoproteins were inserted. Unlike with +ssRNA viruses, naked RNA of –ssRNA viruses are not infectious if delivered into a cell by itself; they have to have RNA polymerase in order to start the cycle of replication.

HIV:

- 2 segments

Influenza

A and B

Viruses:

   - 8 segments

Rotavirus:

   - 11 segments

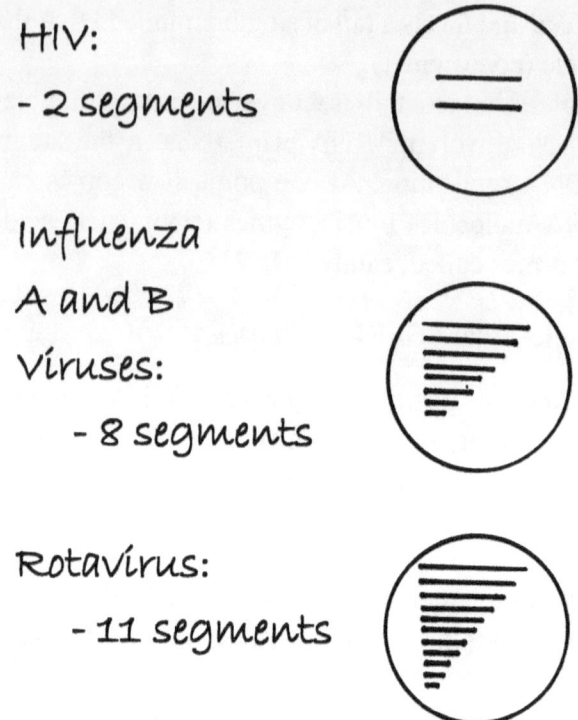

Figure 1.7. Genomes of some RNA viruses

Double-Stranded RNA Viruses

Among double-stranded RNA (dsRNA) viruses, the family of Reoviruses is the most studied. Its members have segmented genomes that encompass ten to twelve pieces of dsRNA. The viral particle that enters the host cell is only partially uncoated; thus, the viral genome remains associated with viral proteins as in −ssRNA viruses. Partial uncoating (stripping) activates enzymes that catalyze the synthesis of the mRNA from each genome fragment. Translation is achieved by the usual cellular machinery, resulting in initiating genome replication. The formed complexes mature into progeny virions.

Retroviruses

Retroviruses are enveloped viruses that belong to the viral family Retroviridae. They synthesize DNA from an RNA template by using reverse transcriptase, which they carry in their capsules. The human immunodeficiency virus (HIV) is a retrovirus. Its capsid contains a material vital for replication:

- A positive-stranded RNA
- A reverse transcriptase with two domains: ribonuclease and polymerase
- An integrase, an enzyme that enables genetic material to be inserted (integrated) into a host cell DNA
- A protease, an enzyme that conducts a proteolysis, a process of hydrolysis of long polypeptides

After the fusion of the viral envelope with the plasma membrane of T lymphocyte, the HIV capsid opens, releasing the HIV genome into the cell's cytoplasm. There, at the polymerase-active side, a single-stranded RNA is transcribed into a RNA-DNA double helix, a hybrid of ssDNA and ssRNA. Afterward, the ribonuclease H breaks this double helix into separate stands. With the help of the polymerase, a complement strand is synthesized, forming double-stranded DNA.

Reverse transcriptase makes five errors per genome, generating multiple antigenic variations.

Then the integrase takes over the process. This enzyme is responsible for the three important events in viral replication:

- It cleaves a tiny piece from each DNA strand, forming "sticky ends" at both ends of the DNA molecule
- It transfers these "sticky ends" of DNA into the nucleus
- It integrates this DNA into the host cell DNA

The proviral DNA either remains in a latent state or actively directs productive infection by, first, inducing the transcription of proviral DNA into the mRNA. The viral mRNA then migrates into the cytoplasm, where polypeptides for a new virus are synthesized. Some of the newly synthesized material has to be processed by the viral protease, which cleaves longer proteins into shorter coproteins. Two vital RNA strands and replication enzymes come together, and coproteins assemble around them in a nucleocapsule. This immature particle takes off, tearing the piece of the cell membrane, which becomes part of the viral envelope. Outside the cell, the virus matures as the protease cleaves some polypeptides to release reverse transcriptase and capsomers. Thus, the virus becomes ready to infect other cells.

Maturation and Release

In most cases, maturation of the viruses occurs within the host cell and includes an assembly during which the genomic nucleic acid is recruited into the capsid, some of which has to be enveloped at the time of release. Some of the envelope proteins are encoded by the viral genes and are incorporated into the plasma membrane of the host cell, in which lipids and carbohydrates are encoded by the genes of the host cell. The envelope wraps around the capsid during the process called budding.

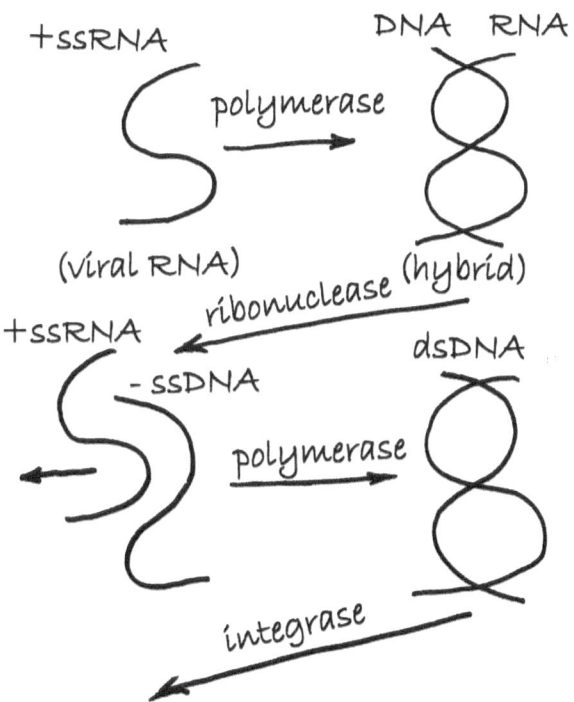

Figure 1.8. Retroviruses: the HIV
replication in a cytoplasm

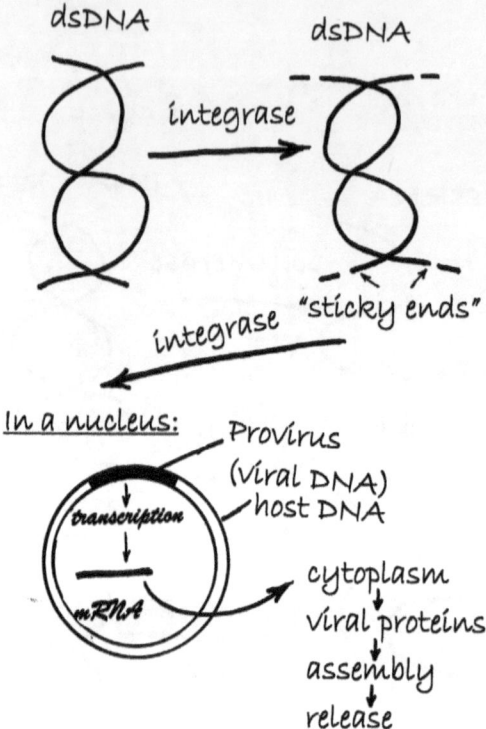

Figure 1.8. (Continued)

The budding occurs in two forms. In the betaretroviruses and the spumaviruses of the Retroviridae, the budding occurs when the fully assembled capsid with the nucleic acid pushes through the plasma membrane. In alpharetroviruses, gammaretroviruses, and lentiviruses, the capsid assembles during budding. Usually, budding does not cause immediate death of the host cell. In some cases, the host survives the process. However, the release of nonenveloped viruses is different. Those viral capsids rupture the host cell membrane, causing immediate destruction and cell death.

CHAPTER II

Enveloped DNA Viruses

Outline

I. Diseases caused by Family Herpesviridae

Genus Herpes *Simplexvirus*

    1. *Herpes simplex virus 1* (HSV-1) infection

    2. *Herpes simplex virus 2* (HSV-2) infection

Genus *Varicellovirus*

    3. Varicella-zoster virus (VZV) infections

Genus *Lymphocryptovirus*

    4. Infectious mononucleosis

    5. Cytomegalovirus (CMV) infection

Genus *Roseolovirus*

    6. Roseola (Sixth Disease)

    7. *Human herpesvirus 7* (HHV-7)

Genus *Rhadinovirus*

    8. *Herpesvirus saimiri* (HHV-8)

II. Diseases caused by Family Poxviridae

    1. Smallpox

    2. *Molluscum contagiosum*

III. Family Hepadnaviridae

    1. Hepatitis B

Family Herpesviridae

The number of cases of human infections caused by the viruses of the family Herpesviridae is enormous. Practically everyone becomes infected with at least some of the herpesviruses; many are not even aware of the infection. These viruses are among the most common and treacherous opportunists among AIDS patients. Herpesviridae contain a linear, double-stranded DNA surrounded by a protein capsid that exhibits icosahedral symmetry (100 nm), which is enclosed in an envelope. The envelope has peplomers, a surface projection. In between the capsid and envelope, there are matrix proteins. The viral genome is large, 120–230 kb. These viruses are ubiquitous. They infect virtually everyone, causing a wide variety of diseases. An interesting attribute of herpesviruses is its ability to switch virion production "on" and "off" and enter an inactive state, establishing a lifelong hidden infection. This type of presence is called latency. The virus remains undetectable in its host cell for long periods of time. The mechanism for controlling latency is unknown.

There are six genera of human pathogens in this family of viruses:

- Herpes simplex viruses
- Varicella-zoster viruses
- Epstein-Barr viruses
- Cytomegaloviruses
- Human herpes 6 and 7 viruses
- *Human herpesvirus 8*

There is little DNA homology among these human herpesviruses except for 50% homology between the herpes simplex-1 and the herpes simplex-2.

Genus Herpes Simplex Viruses

Table 2.1
Properties of HSVs

Alternative names of HSV infection: cold sores, fever blisters

Size: 150–200 nm in diameter

Envelope: from nuclear membrane and from membrane of Golgi complex

Capsid: icosahedral (16 surfaces), 162 capsomers

Genome: two covalently linked segments dsDNA (cyclize in preparation for replication), 152 kbp, ~74 genes

Target cell type: mucoepithelia

Inclusions: form prominent inclusions in the nucleus

Latency: neuron

Transmission: direct contact

Diseases: herpes, genital herpes, pharyngitis, pneumonia; in neonates: meningitis, encephalitis, blinding keratitis, disseminated necrosis of the skin

Therapy: acyclovir

The clinical response to the infection with herpes simplex viruses (HSVs)—commonly known as herpes—is ordinarily a mild vesicular eruption of the skin or mucous membranes. The eruption is both grossly and microscopically similar to varicella and zoster; however, the viruses are unrelated antigenically and biologically (different host range). An inactive state of HSV occurs in sensory neurons. Control of transcription is likely to be a central process in the molecular interactions between HSV and its host cells. The host functions are also likely to play a role in the repression of viral gene expression. HSV does not display its antigens on the surfaces of neurons. Consequently, cytotoxic T cells cannot recognize and kill infected neurons. A latent infection forms a reservoir of the virus for recurrent outbreaks and transmission to other individuals.

Viral replication can be reactivated by such immunosuppression stimuli as stress, sunlight, change of temperature, menstruation, etc. As the viruses migrate from the neurons to epithelial cells, where they once again replicate, a recurrence of symptoms occurs. Herpes simplexviruses are categorized into two types:

- *Herpes simplex virus 1* (HSV-1 or oral herpes)
- *Herpes simplex virus 2* (HSV-2 or genital herpes)

Both HSV-1 and HSV-2 can infect many regions in the body, depending on the type of contact. In HSV-2, the infected person may have sores around the genitals or rectum. Although HSV-2 sores may occur in other locations, these sores usually are found below the waist. Both HSV-1 and HSV-2 can be spread even if characteristic blisters are not present.

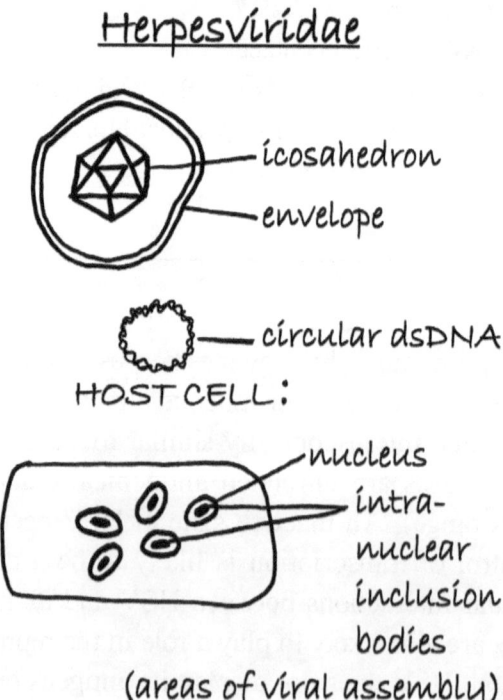

Figure 2.1. Herpesviridae: viral architecture
and inclusion bodies within a host cell

Herpes simplex virus 1 Infection

Most commonly, herpes simplex type 1 causes sores around the mouth and lips. Colloquial names are fever blisters and cold sores. HSV type 1 (HSV-1) is ordinarily associated with primary infections of the orofacial area. Latent HSV genomes reside in the nuclei of neuron cell bodies in trigeminal ganglia. HSV-1 can cause genital herpes, but it more commonly causes infections of the mouth and lips. HSV-1 infection of the genitals can be caused by oral-genital or genital-genital contact with a person who has HSV-1 infection. Genital HSV-1 outbreaks recur less regularly than genital HSV-2 outbreaks. HSV-1, which is transmitted through oral secretions or sores on the skin, can be spread through kissing or sharing objects such as toothbrushes or eating utensils. No specific control measures are recommended.

HSV-1 is capable of causing HSV pneumonia triggered by formation of HSV vesicles in the distal airways. Patients with HSV-pneumonia who have not received specific anti-HSV therapy usually improve slowly over a prolonged time. Therapy with acyclovir results in prompt improvement of the patient's hypoxemia.

Cultures of respiratory secretions from patients with HSV pneumonia are usually negative. The diagnosis is ordinarily confirmed by a cytology report that indicates the presence of the cytopathic effects of HSV-1 and the presence of ground-glass-appearing nuclei along with intranuclear-inclusion bodies. The nuclear chromatin is displaced to the edge of the cell nucleus, giving it an "owl's eye" appearance.

Herpes simplex virus 2 Infection

Herpes simplex virus 2 infection, or HSV-2 infection, is the most common sexually transmitted disease in the USA. It is commonly known as genital herpes. HSV-2 is ordinarily associated with genital infections and a latent infection in the sacral ganglia.

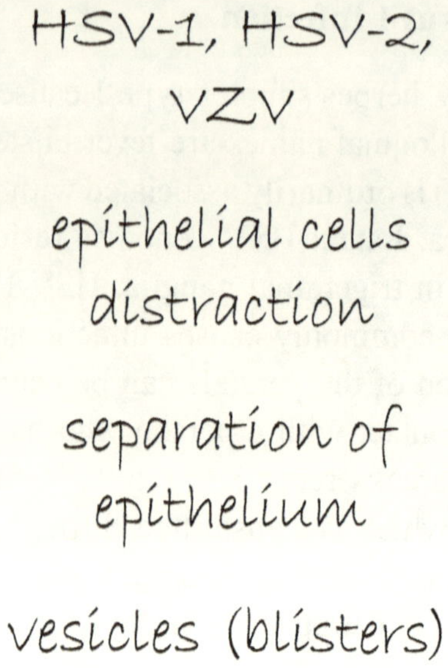

HSV-1, HSV-2, VZV

epithelial cells
distraction

separation of
epithelium

vesicles (blisters)

Figure 2.2. HSV-1, HSV-2, and VZV pathogenicity

Signs and symptoms. The infection causes recurrent and painful genital sores, but the symptoms can often be very innocuous or may be mistaken for insect bites or another skin condition. Therefore, some infected individuals are unaware of their condition. During the primary episode, a first outbreak, a clinical presentation can be quite pronounced. Flulike symptoms, including fever and swollen glands, may manifest with a second crop of sores. People diagnosed with a first episode of genital herpes can expect to have over five other symptomatic recurrences within a year. The characteristic lesion is a fluid-filled vesicle that erupts and becomes an ulcer. These open sores are teeming with viruses and are very infectious. They occur anywhere on the penis in men and on the vagina, vulva, and cervix in women. The anus, perineum, buttocks, and thighs of either sex may also be ulcerated. The lesions are frequently painful but sometimes undetected. People with painless lesions are often unaware that they are infected and shed the virus until notified of a subsequent outbreak in a sex partner. Over time, these recurrences usually decrease in frequency.

Diagnosis. HSV infections can be diagnosed clinically during the outbreaks or between outbreaks by antibodies' detection.

Incubation period. The first outbreak usually occurs within two weeks after the virus is transmitted. The sores ordinarily heal within two to four weeks.

Sequelae. HSV can cause serious diseases such as neonatal disseminated herpes, viral meningitis, viral encephalitis, blinding keratitis, and disseminated necrosis of the skin or other potentially fatal disorders. The neonatal infections are acquired during normal delivery through the birth canal of a woman with open lesions. Also, genital herpes infection has been associated with an increased risk for HIV-1 infection. Long-term neurological symptoms have occasionally been associated with HSV infection.

Transmission. The virus is most commonly transmitted when active herpetic lesions are present in the genital area. The vesicle fluid has HSV in high concentrations but can be transmitted from skin that does not appear to have sores. The virus can also be shed in urine and genital secretions when no lesions are present.

Treatment. Genital herpes is an incurable disease. Most of the time, the blister outbreaks can be controlled with an antiviral drug called acyclovir, sold as Zovirax, Zirgan, and Valtrex. It is a potent inhibitor against both HSV-1 and HSV-2 and is virtually nontoxic to humans.

Epidemiology. The estimated total number of people aged fifteen to forty-nine years who are living with HSV-2 worldwide in 2003 was 536 million. According to that estimation, more women than men were infected, with an estimated 315 million infected women compared to 221 million infected men. The number infected increased with age and peaked in the age stratum thirty-five to thirty-nine after which it declined slightly. Overall, Americans are infected with the STD at 16%, which are about one out of six individuals.

At least five hundred thousand join their ranks each year. The CDC has released data showing that African Americans currently have a 39.2% infection rate compared to European Americans, who have a 12.3% infection rate. Upward of 48% of African American women are infected with *Herpes simplex virus 2*. HSV-2 prevalence is nearly twice as high among women (21%) as men (11.5%) and more than three times higher among African Americans (39%) than whites (12%). In Western Europe, the HSV-2 prevalence is around 18% among women and 13% among men. In sub-Saharan Africa, the prevalence reaches a maximum of 70% among women and around 55% among men.

Prevention. The people with symptoms that might be caused by the virus should be tested by their physicians. They should abstain from sexual activity with uninfected partners when lesions or other symptoms of herpes are present. Sex partners of infected persons should be advised that they may become infected. Condoms should be used to decrease the risk of infection. Use of acyclovir halves the likelihood of transmission to a sexual partner.

Cultures. The virus has a wide host range and can infect rabbits, guinea pigs, mice, hamsters, rats, and the chorioallantois of the embryonated egg. The chorioallantoic membrane is particularly susceptible to infection; lesions become obvious in one to two days and reach their maximum in three to four days. They are small white raised plaques, and their number is directly proportionate to the concentration of virus particles. The virus also grows readily in tissue culture, producing typical inclusions; inclusion body formation is followed by necrosis of cells, a cytopathic effect. Human amnion or rabbit kidney cultures are the cells of choice.

Genus Varicellovirus

Members of this genus, besides causing various diseases in monkeys, horses, and pigs, infect humans, causing chicken pox, which later during life cause an outbreak of shingles. The genome of the etiological agent of this disease, varicella zoster virus (VZV), is strikingly similar to the genome of HSV. Thus, sixty-four out of sixty-nine genes are homologous to HSV. Moreover, like HSV, VZV establishes lifelong latent infection in sensory ganglia and, during outbreaks, produces the vesicles filled with a fluid that contains large amounts of free, ready-to-spread viruses.

Chicken Pox and Shingles

Table 2.2
Properties of the Varicella Zoster Virus (VZV)

Alternative name: *Human herpesvirus 3* (HHV-3)

Size: 180–200 nm

Envelope: from nuclear membrane, Golgi apparatus, endoplasmic reticulum, cytoplasmic membrane

Capsid: icosahedral (16 surfaces), 162 capsomers, 100–110 nm in diameter

Genome: dsDNA, linear (cyclize in preparation for replication), ~125 kbp, 69 genes of which all but five are homologous to genes in HSV

Target cell type: epithelial cells, reticuloendothelial system

Inclusions: form prominent inclusions in the nucleus

Latency: neuron

Transmission: direct contact or respiratory route

Diseases: chicken pox and shingles

Therapy: acyclovir, varicella zoster immunoglobulin (VZIG)

Vaccine: attenuated virus (for chicken pox—children and adults without evidence of immunity); attenuated virus (for shingles—adults age 60 and over)

The VZV causes two different diseases, known as chicken pox (varicella) and shingles (zoster). Those two diseases represent two phases of activity of the VZV, which is morphologically identical to the herpes simplex virus. It is characterized by a vascular eruption of the skin and mucous membrane. The target cells of VZV are epithelial cells. Under viral attack, they swell and balloon, and the accumulation of tissue fluids in the epithelial tissue results in vesicle formation. A painful condition affecting nerve fibers and skin is called postherpetic neuralgia. In the blister-like lesions of the skin in either disease, there are typical reddish inclusion bodies in the nuclei of the injured epithelial cells. The virus is plentiful in the vesicle fluid of either disease. The moist crusts of injured skin are infectious, whereas the dry ones are not. In rare instances, when the patient dies of disseminated varicella, giant cells are found in many organs of the body.

After the primary infection, the virus remains latent in the sensory ganglia. It reactivates upon weakening of the cellular immune system due to various conditions, erupting from sensory neurons and infecting the corresponding skin tissue. The factors involved in the neuronal invasion and the establishment of latency are still elusive.

Signs and symptoms. Chicken pox is a highly contagious but mild disease of childhood. It manifests with malaise and fever followed within a day or two by the sudden outbreak of a vesicular rash distributed ordinarily centripetally (meaning with a concentration on the trunk) unlike in vesicular eruptions in smallpox where crops of skin lesions have centrifugal distribution (meaning on the face and limbs). Chicken pox lesions may also appear in the buccal and pharyngeal mucosa. In contrast to smallpox, all stages of papules, vesicles, and crusts in chicken pox develop simultaneously and may be seen at one time. Intense itching tempts the child to scratch the lesions, leading to a bacterial superinfection and permanent scarring. Primary chicken pox of adults is a more serious illness than the primary infection of children.

Chicken Pox
(varicella)
-occurs in epidemics
Not to be confused with:
Varicella = chicken pox =
= Herpesviridae
Variola = smallpox =
= Poxviridae

Figure 2.3. Varicella calcification and pathogenicity

Signs and symptoms of shingles. Shingles is a sporadic, incapacitating disease of adults that is rare in children. Malaise and fever are soon followed by severe pain in the area of the skin or the mucosa supplied by one or more groups of sensory nerves. The inflammatory reaction that typically is found in the dorsal nerve roots and ganglia occasionally spreads to the anterior horn cells, resulting in a paralysis that is usually temporary. Within a few days after the onset, a crop of vesicles appear over the skin supplied by the affected nerves, usually on the trunk, head, and neck. Second attacks are not common and do not necessarily occur on the same dermatome.

Diagnosis. Diagnosis is made on the clinical appearance. If the symptoms are not straightforward in some patients, such as those who are immunosuppressed, diagnostic tests can be performed. The most common are immunofluorescence assay and PCR.

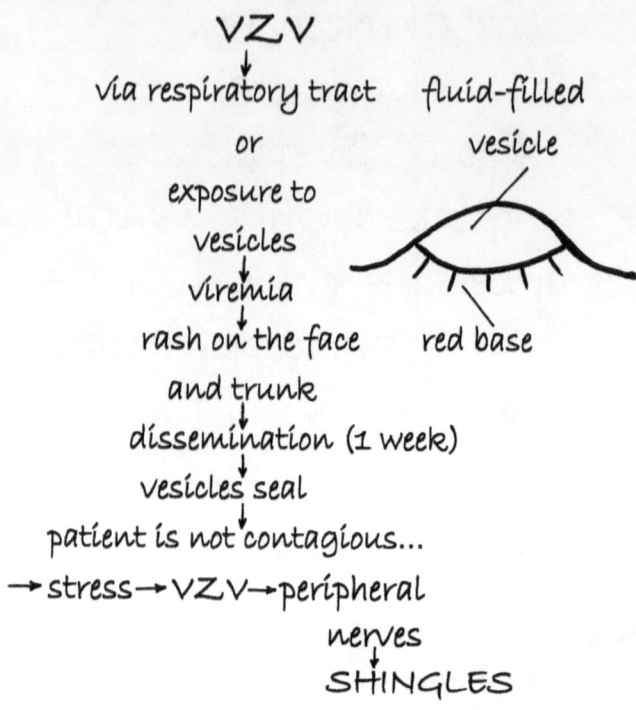

VZV
↓
via respiratory tract   fluid-filled
or   vesicle
exposure to
vesicles
↓
viremia
rash on the face   red base
and trunk
↓
dissemination (1 week)
↓
vesicles seal
↓
patient is not contagious...
→ stress → VZV → peripheral
nerves
↓
SHINGLES

Figure 2.3. (Continued)

Incubation period. The incubation period of chicken pox is ten to twenty-one days.

Sequelae. Complications are unusual, except in adults in whom severe pneumonitis is sometimes accompanied by hepatitis, which may supervene a few days after the rash appears. Encephalitis is rare (1 in 1,000).

The most common complication in otherwise healthy children is a bacterial infection of the skin lesions. Reye's syndrome is an occasional severe complication of chicken pox. A few days after the initial infection is retreated, the patient persistently vomits and exhibits signs of brain dysfunction. Fatty degeneration of the liver, coma, and death can follow. Virtually, Reye's syndrome affects only children and teenagers. The primary adult infection with VZV can lead to male sterility, acute liver failure, and other complications.

Transmission. The transmission of VZV can either be via direct contact or by the respiratory route. The port of entry may be the respiratory tract, the oropharynx, or the conjunctiva. The virus replicates at the primary inoculation site and then disseminates via the lymphatics and the bloodstream.

Treatment. A few studies indicate that antiviral medications decrease the duration of symptoms and the likelihood of postherpetic neuralgia, especially when initiated within two days of the onset of the rash. Other medications, including valacyclovir, penciclovir, and famciclovir, are also available.

Epidemiology. VZV has a worldwide distribution, but infection is almost universal in temperate regions. In adults, zoster occurs sporadically and without seasonal prevalence while, in contrast, chicken pox is one of the common epidemic diseases of childhood. It is more common in winter and spring than in summer. In tropical regions, only about half of the population contracts chicken pox. In contrast to HSV-1 and HSV-2, VZV reactivates infrequently.

Prevention. Vaccines are available for prevention of both chicken pox and shingles. The chicken pox vaccine was licensed for use in the USA in 1995. The vaccine is made from weakened varicella virus.

Cultures. VZV propagates in cultures of human embryonic tissue with the production of typical intranuclear inclusion bodies. Supernatant fluids from such infected cultures have contained a complement-fixing antigen but have been free of infective virus. Fluids harvested from infected thyroid cells have yielded the infectious virus. It has not been propagated in laboratory animals.

Genus Lymphocryptovirus

The Epstein-Barr virus and the cytomegalovirus belong to the genus *Lymphocryptovirus* of the Herpesviridae family.

Infectious Mononucleosis

Table 2.3
Properties of Epstein-Barr Virus

Alternative name: *Human herpesvirus 4* (HHV-4)

Size: 120–150 nm in diameter

Envelope: plasma membrane

Capsid: icosahedral

Genome: linear (cyclize in preparation for replication) dsDNA, 172 kbp

Target cell type: B cells, epithelial cells; occasionally, T cells and NK cells

Latency: B cells

Transmission: saliva

Diseases: infectious mononucleosis, pneumonia, Burkitt's lymphoma, nasopharyngeal carcinoma, Hodgkin's disease, and T cell lymphomas

---

Infectious mononucleosis is the most common viral infection in humans that might be either very mild, even asymptomatic, or can cause a debilitating illness with sequelae. Infectious mononucleosis was first named glandular fever in the 1880s by German doctors. Informal names are the *kissing disease* and *everybody's virus* infection. The causative agent is one of the most common viruses called Epstein-Barr virus (EBV). It is named after Tony Epstein and Yvonne Barr, who first described the virus in tumor cells from patients with Burkitt's lymphoma in 1964. Like all other members of the family, EBV capsid is enveloped. Virions are spherical or pleomorphic. Its genome is not segmented and consists of a single molecule of double-stranded DNA that had been fully sequenced. In mononucleosis, EBV infects the human B cells by first binding to the complement receptor (C3d) on the cells. Inside the cell, EBV prevents it from undergoing a normal life cycle. Thus, it transforms cells into malignant (cancer) cells passing on copies of EBV DNA to their progeny. It remains in the latent state as multiple copies of circular DNA (cDNA). With its activation and multiplication, infected cells burst, releasing the viruses for their new journey. A fascinating attribute of this process is that the cancer cells suddenly disappear with a resolution of the mononucleosis. Perhaps the immune system destroys the infecting virus along with abnormal B cells.

Most people who become infected in childhood trigger few signs and symptoms or no symptoms at all. If the initial infection is delayed until adolescents, EBV causes infectious mononucleosis in about 35%–50% of those infected.

Signs and symptoms. It takes from four to six weeks for the first symptoms to occur. Symptoms may include sore throat (82%), malaise (57%), headache (51%), anorexia (21%), myalgias (20%), chills (16%), nausea (12%), abdominal discomfort (9%), cough (5%), arthralgias (2%), very painful pharyngitis (84%), fever (76%), hepatomegaly (12%), jaundice (9%), and rash (10%). Many have enlarged lymph nodes (94%) and splenomegaly, an enlarged spleen (52%), as the B cells multiply. The symptoms rarely last for more than four months; if they persist for more than six, the infection is considered chronic. In this case, the patient's condition should be investigated to determine if the illness meets the chronic fatigue syndrome, ruling out other causes of a chronic illness.

Sequelae. An enlarged spleen in patients with an EBV infection is prone to rupture; therefore, patients with *mono* are advised not to play contact sports since a ruptured spleen can cause a medical emergency. Other complications are rare but include jaundice, skin rashes, pancreatitis, seizures, encephalitis, Burkitt's lymphoma (BL), nasopharyngeal carcinoma (NPC), Hodgkin's disease, and T cell lymphomas.

BL is a childhood malignancy that occurs predominantly in places in Africa and New Guinea with a high incidence of malaria. The tumors arise in lymph nodes, often in submandibular nodes. If not treated, the disease is fatal. With treatment, the majority of patients can survive. One of the recent hypotheses explain an association of the disease with malaria because of the expansion of germinal centers that result from malaria infection. This leads to the increased incidence of lymphomas.

NPC is also worldwide but has a much higher incidence in Southeast Asia, in Eskimos, and among some populations in Northern and Eastern Africa. Studies suggest that both genetic and environmental factors are important for the higher incidence in these populations.

Hodgkin's disease is another form of malignant lymphoma. It often strikes young adults, although there is a peak in incidence after the age of forty-five. Like diseases described above, it is worldwide, though more common in developed countries. Little is known about the process by which the EBV infects T cells and causes tumors. Immunocompromised people are at greatly increased risk for the development of lymphomas caused by EBV.

Diagnoses. Diagnoses are usually based on the clinical symptoms of the disease and the age of the patient. When children are infected with EBV, symptoms are undistinguishable or mild. When infections occur during adolescence or young adulthood, it causes infectious mononucleosis 35%–50% of the time.

Serological tests determine an elevated leukocytes count (complete blood count), especially atypical ones, and a positive reaction on a monospot test, a form of the heterophile antibody test that rapidly identifies mononucleosis caused by EBV. Heterophile stands for reactivity with proteins across species lines; the presence of heterophile antibodies leads to the formation of agglutinates, blood clumps in the mixture of serum from the infected individual combined with cow's and horse's erythrocytes and guinea pigs' kidney stroma. Many EBV-infected people develop heterophile antibodies a week after the onset of symptoms, but some people infected with EBV never do.

A monospot test that comes in a kit helps to diagnose a recent EBV infection and is commercially available. The test sensitivity is moderate, 70%–90% sensitive, but its specificity is high, 96%–100% specific. If test results are positive, it confirms an EBV infection, but if the test comes out negative, it does not necessary rule out an infection being present. This test does not give a positive result during the incubation period of the illness nor after active infection is subsided despite the fact that the virus may still be in the cells. False positive results on EBV infection may be obtained in patients with hepatitis, rubella, systemic lupus erythematosus, leukemia, lymphoma, or certain gastrointestinal cancers.

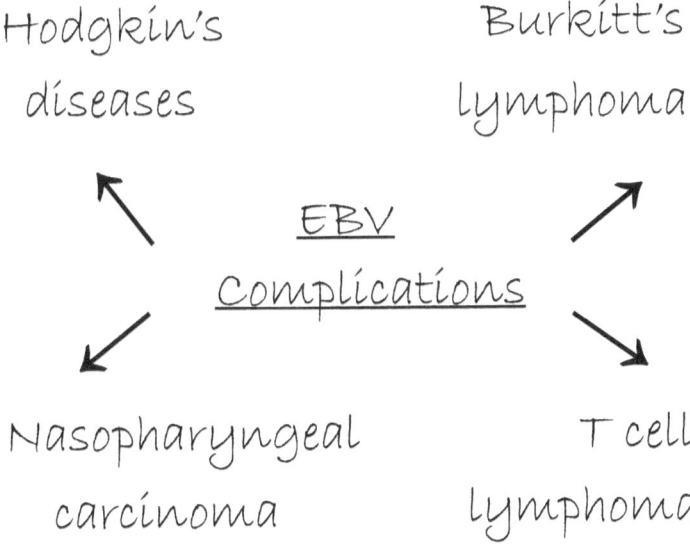

Figure 2.4. EBV complications

If a person is symptomatic but the monospot test is negative, the antibody test could be used. The EBV antibody test is a series of tests that can detect different types of antibodies against EBV to determine whether the patient was infected with EBV recently or sometime in the past. IgM antibodies are detected when mono is in its active phase. IgG antibodies are found later when the patient is starting to feel better. There is also a molecular test that measures EBV DNA. This test is usually used in monitoring EBV in patients with Burkitt's lymphoma, Hodgkin's lymphoma, or a posttransplant lymphoproliferative disease.

Transmission. Transmission occurs through saliva; transmission through air or blood does not normally occur. The primary reservoir of the EBVs is healthy people who carry the virus in their saliva. People who have been exposed to EBV are not at risk of developing infectious mononucleosis. When adults who had never been infected with EBV in childhood become infected with EBV, the most common signs of the infection are liver enlargement and jaundice.

Epidemiology. The virus occurs worldwide. In the USA, 95% of adults between the ages thirty-five and forty have been infected, so true outbreaks of infectious mononucleosis are extremely rare. In the underdeveloped countries, infectious mononucleosis is not as common as in developed countries because most people become infected with EBV during early childhood, when symptoms of the disease are minimal or asymptomatic.

Treatment. There is no medication against EBVs; therefore, care is largely supportive. Radiotherapy and chemotherapy are utilized in treating EBV-associated malignancies.

Prevention. Since the carriers of the virus are healthy people and there is a lack of vaccine, the transmission is almost impossible to prevent.

Cultures. EBV grows readily in B cells cultures. The receptor used to enter B cells is a protein called CD21. Attempts to infect epithelial cells in culture have not been successful, though it is thought that the differentiation status of the epithelial cell is important for the expression of the full lytic cycle.

Historical reference. The term *infectious mononucleosis* was first coined in 1920. In 1968, this virus was linked to infectious mononucleosis and other clinical syndromes. In 1970, it had been shown to immobilize B lymphocytes.

Cytomegalovirus Infection

Table 2.4
Properties of CMV

Alternative name: *Human herpesvirus 5* (HHV-5)

Envelop: from plasma membrane

Capsid: icosahedral, 162 capsomers

Genome: linear (cyclize in preparation for replication) dsDNA, ~235 kbp

Target cell type: epithelia, monocytes, lymphocytes

Inclusion bodies: cytomegalic inclusions, prominent in enlarged cell nucleus and cytoplasm

Latency: monocytes, lymphocytes, and possibly others

Transmission: direct contact, blood transfusions, transplantation, sexual contact

Diseases: opportunistic infection in organ transplant recipients and in patients with AIDS, cytomegalic inclusion disease, and microcephaly in neonates

Cytopathy: formation of cytomegalic cells

Therapy: ganciclovir, foscarnet, intravenous immunoglobulin (IVIG)

Human cytomegalovirus (HCMV) is a member of the enveloped herpesvirus family and a widespread pathogen that causes diseases in immunologically immature or compromised individuals. Cytomegalovirus (CMV) infection is virtually in all immunocompetent individuals. About 80% of adults in the United States have antibodies against CMV, yet the virus rarely causes disease but persists for long periods as a latent or chronic infection of salivary and other glands. If reactivation of the CMV occurs during pregnancy, it can cross the placenta and cause congenital disease. About 0.5% of all infants in the United States have congenital CMV. It is the most common viral cause of mental retardation and multiple birth defects. Many of the infected children die shortly before or after birth. In adults, the viral transmission occurs through the contact of the mucosal surface with body secretions that contain the CMV. Approximately 90% of the population in developing countries is seropositive by the age of six years as compared to less than 30% in the United States and Western Europe. CMV is a major opportunistic infection in organ transplant recipients and in patients with AIDS.

Cytopathy. The disease is characterized by production of cytomegalic cells. Those cells are greatly swollen, with an enlarged nucleus distended by basophilic or sometimes eosinophilic intranuclear inclusions. They are separated by a nonstaining halo ("owl's eye") from the nuclear membrane. Their small inclusions may be present in the cell's cytoplasm of salivary glands, in the lungs, liver, pancreas, kidneys, endocrine glands, and occasionally, in the brain.

Prevention. Organs harvested for transplantation can be made safe by treatment with monoclonal antibodies against CMV. For CMV-seronegative organ transplant recipients, organs from CMV-seronegative donors should be used if possible. There is no vaccine against CMV.

Genus Roseolovirus

Roseolovirus is genetically related to CMV. It encompasses *Human herpesvirus 6* (HHV-6) and *Human herpesvirus 7* (HHV-7). HHV-6 is a ubiquitous human pathogen infecting over 95% of the population by the age of two years and, as with other herpesviruses reactivation of HHV-6, can be present with severe complications in immunocompromised individuals.

Roseola (Sixth Disease)

Table 2.5
Properties of *Human herpesvirus 6* (HHV-6)

Alternative names: *Human herpesvirus 6* (HHV-6)

Envelope: plasma membrane

Capsid: icosahedral, 162 capsomers

Genome: linear (cyclize in preparation for replication) dsDNA, 159 kbp

Target cell type: lymphocytes, especially CD4+ T cells

Transmission: aerosol, oral secretions

Diseases: roseola, a childhood rash disease

Diagnosis: ordinarily diagnosed clinically

Symptoms: high fever followed by macular body rush

Therapy: supportive care

Prevention: there is no vaccine available

Roseola (exanthema subitum, roseola infantum) is a common and mild disease of childhood that ordinarily affects six-month-olds to three-year-olds. It is characterized by a sudden onset of high fever (105°F) that causes convulsions. After several days, the fever subsides and a short-lived red rash appears, ordinarily on the chest and abdomen. It could be present for as short as a few hours or for as long as five days. More severe symptoms or neurological complications occur only rarely. Primary infections in adults with *Human herpesvirus 6* (HHV-6) are uncommon because of the immunity that had been developed from the childhood infection; however, when it occurs, the symptoms are more serious. The virus is probably transmitted by oral secretions. Over 95% of the population is infected with HHV-6 by age 3.

Historical reference. HHV-6 was first isolated in 1986 from the peripheral blood of patients with lymphoproliferative disorders and AIDS.

Human herpesvirus 7

Extensive research on HHV-6 led to the discovery of its closest sibling – a human herpes virus 7 (HHV-7), in 1990. It had been recovered first from T-cells of a healthy donor and from a patient with CFS/ME. As with HHV-6, 95% of population is infected with HHV-7. Over 75% are infected before six years of age. There is no childhood disease or a definable syndrome that is associated with an acute HHV-7 infection.

Genus Rhadinovirus

Rhadinoviruses are a genus of herpesviruses that include the simian virus best known as *Herpesvirus saimiri* (HVS), also known as Kaposi's sarcoma–associated herpesvirus (KSHV) or simply *Human herpesvirus 8* (HHV-8).

Herpesvirus Saimiri

Table 2.6
Properties of *Herpesvirus saimiri*

Alternative names: *Human herpesvirus 8* (HHV-8)
Envelope: plasma membrane
Capsid: circular dsDNA (linear during replication), icosadeltahedral lattice with 20 faces, 125 nm in diameter
Genome: linear dsDNA (circular in the host cell), 170 kbp (Rene et al.) 270 kbp (Moore et al.)
Target cell type: epithelial cells, endothelial cells, keratinocytes, macrophages, and B cells
Latency: Unknown
Transmission: saliva, sexual intercourse, blood, and transplant-related transmission
Diseases: Kaposi's sarcoma, Castleman's disease

Herpesvirus saimiri virus belongs to the genus *Rhadinovirus*. It causes fatal T-lymphoproliferative disorders in nonhuman primates, while in a natural host, a squirrel monkey, it persists in the T lymphocytes without causing any apparent disease. *Herpesvirus saimiri* is also known by the following names:

- Saimiriine herpesvirus type 2
- *Human herpesvirus 8* (HHV-8)
- Kaposi's sarcoma–associated herpesvirus (KSHV)

The virus is also responsible for infections in humans, which include the following:

- Kaposi's sarcoma, a cancer that causes patches of abnormal tissue to grow under the skin or in the mucous membranes, in the lining of the mouth, nose, throat, and anus. Today, it is the most common malignancy seen in HIV-infected patients. The Kaposi's sarcoma cells resemble blood vessels, and its lesions usually appear on the skin as raised blotches or nodules that may be purple, red, or brown. Before the AIDS epidemic, Kaposi's sarcoma was seen mainly in elderly Italian and Jewish men.
- Primary effusion lymphoma (PEL) is a rare HIV-associated non-Hodgkin's lymphoma (NHL) that accounts for approximately 4% of all HIV-associated NHL.
- Castleman's disease, a rare lymphoproliferative disorder that involves a single lymph node (unicentric Castleman disease) or can be a systemic (multicentric Castleman disease) infection. It is also known as giant lymph node hyperplasia and angiofollicular lymph node hyperplasia. The disease is similar to cancers of the lymphatic system (lymphomas), though it is not considered a cancer. However, it is still linked to lymphomas.

Historical reference. The disease was previously described by the Hungarian dermatologist Moritz Kaposi in 1872. HHV-8 was first characterized in HIV-infected patients with Kaposi's sarcoma in 1994. Subsequently, HHV-8 was found to be associated with many other disorders, including Kaposi's sarcoma, PEL, and Castleman's disease. The introduction of highly active antiretroviral therapy (HAART) in the late 1990s has decreased the overall incidence of AIDS-related NHL.

Family Poxviridae

Poxviridae are a very large family of unusual dsDNA viruses that infect mammals, birds, and insects. Unlike the rest of DNA viruses, they replicate their DNA in the cytoplasm, not the nucleus. They require a virion-associated transcriptase in order to make the various viral enzymes to synthesize all their nucleic acids. They do not use cellular polymerases, ligases, and other enzymes since they are located in the nucleus. *Poxviridae* direct the synthesis of their own envelopes while other viruses simply modify human cell membranes. Only two human poxviruses are known, variola or the smallpox virus, a member of *Orthopox* genus, and molluscum contagiosum virus (MCV), the only member of the genus *Molluscipoxvirus*. However, a number of mammalian poxviruses can cause a limited and abortive natural infections of humans as well as the avian poxviruses can infect humans under experimental conditions. Those poxviruses have been used as agents for vaccination against virulent human viruses. Poxviruses are exceptional among DNA viruses because they replicate in the cytoplasm, unlike the rest of the DNA viruses that replicate in the nucleus.

Smallpox (Variola)

Table 2.7
Properties of Smallpox Virus

Virion: brick shaped, 350 × 270 nm
Envelope: either cell membrane or newly synthesized (?)
Capsid: brick shaped; has a biconcave core and two lateral bodies
Genome: circular dsDNA, 130–375 kbp
Target cell type: epithelial cells and lymphocytes
Transmission: direct contact through skin abrasion
Therapy: immediate vaccination after exposure
Eradication: by *Vaccinia virus* immunization
Diseases: smallpox (variola), monkeypox

Smallpox, which also previously known as variola major, is an acute infectious disease characterized by severe systemic involvement and a single crop of skin lesions that proceeds through macular, papular, vesicular, and pustular stages over a period of five to ten days. A mild form, variola minor, is also known. Variola minor was endemic in Africa and the America and coexisted with variola major. *Vaccinia virus* is a related poxvirus, attenuated for man and had long been in used as the first live virus vaccine. The smallpox virus is one of the largest and most resilient viruses known as it can live apart from its host for decades.

The smallpox virus and *Vaccinia virus* can withstand drying for a month, even when held at room temperature. They endure lower temperatures for years. In the moist state, the virus is destroyed at 60°C for ten minutes, but in the dry state, it can resist 100°C for five to ten minutes. One medical researcher published a paper in which he recommended that archaeologists who work on mummies should be vaccinated against smallpox.

<u>Poxviridae</u>

- Replicate in cytoplasm (!)
- no animal reservoir

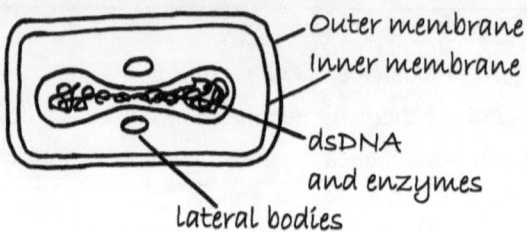

Smallpox Skin Lesions

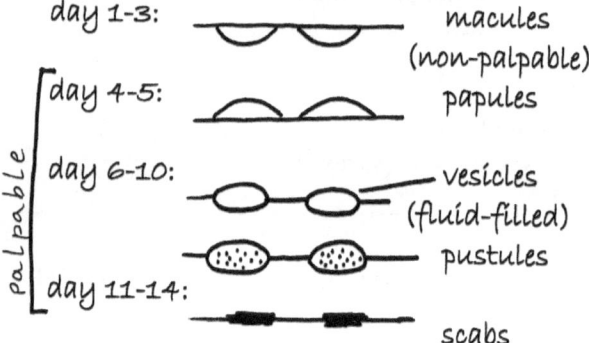

Figure 2.5. Architecture of Poxviridae
and smallpox skin lesions

Virus-infected cells:

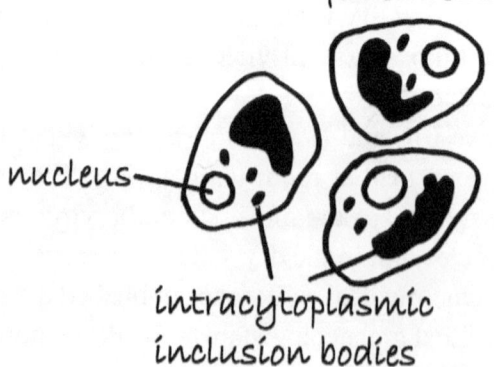

Figure 2.6. Inclusion bodies of *Vaccinia virus*

Acids (pH 3) destroy the virus within an hour. Phenol (1%) has little effect at 4°C but inactivates the virus at 37°C in twenty-four hours. Alcohol in 50% concentration or potassium permanganate in 0.01% concentration destroys the virus within one hour at room temperature.

Signs and symptoms. The growth of the virus in the epidermal layers of the skin and mucous membranes causes lesions.

Diagnosis. The elementary bodies of the smallpox virus may be seen microscopically within cells of a stained preparation of scrapings taken from a lesion.

Incubation period. The incubation period is about twelve days. The onset may be gradual or sudden.

Sequelae. Skin pustules may become contaminated, usually with staphylococci, sometimes leading to a number of bacterial complications such as osteomyelitis and septic joints. In severe cases, the rash is hemorrhagic. The mortality rate varies from 5% with a discrete rash to over 40% with a confluent rash.

Transmission. Smallpox is one of the most highly communicable diseases. The portal of entry of the variola virus is through the mucous membranes of the upper respiratory tract. It can be acquired through a droplet, by airborne route, or contact transmission by hand contact with the pustules. During the incubation period, the virus may propagate in the lymphoid and other tissues. Since infected individuals have no open lesions on the mucosal surface during incubation, they are not infectious during this period. The skin lesion follows the localization of the virus in the epidermis via the bloodstream.

Treatment. Vaccinia immune globulin (VIG) should be given as soon as possible after exposure. After clinical signs of smallpox are evident, VIG is of no value. Antibiotics have no effect in the early stages of smallpox but may be of value in preventing secondary bacterial infection in the pustular stage.

Epidemiology. WHO declared in 1980 that because of effective vaccination, smallpox was eradicated from human population. It is thought that the last victim of a natural case of smallpox was one who had recovered from variola minor in 1977 in Somalia, Africa. The eradication of smallpox was possible because there were no animal host reservoirs for the disease. Today only two sites maintain the smallpox virus in their facilities, one in the USA and one in Russia.

Prevention. Smallpox vaccination is not an innocuous procedure and is no longer recommended for universal usage.

Cultures. The host range of the variola virus is restricted to man and monkeys.

Unlike the *Vaccinia virus*, it cannot be propagated in rabbits or mice. However, it grows readily on the chorioallantoic membrane of the ten- to twelve-day-old chick embryo. It produces characteristic small white lesions that are different from the large vaccinia lesions, having central depressions due to necrosis. The morphologic character of the lesion produced on the chick membrane used to be used for rapid identification of the variola virus in clinical specimens. The vaccinia virus grows readily in cultures of chick embryo or primate cells, producing necrosis of the cells. Monkey kidney cell cultures are much more sensitive than rabbit skin in vivo.

Molluscum Contagiosum

Molluscum contagiosum virus (MCV), a brick-shaped virus, causes small benign skin lesions in children and young adults and a more extensive disease only when there is a concurrent immunodeficiency such as AIDS.

Signs and symptoms. The benign lesions of this disease are small pink -wart-like tumors with nipple-like indentations on the face, arms, back, and buttocks. Cells in the nodule are greatly hypertrophied and contain large hyaline acidophilic cytoplasmic masses called molluscum bodies. Individual molluscum lesions may resolve on their own in six to eight weeksor in two to three months. However, due to autoinoculation, the disease may propagate with a range of durations from six months to five years.

Diagnosis. Diagnosis is made on the clinical appearance and confirmed by excisional biopsy.

Incubation period. The incubation period in human volunteers has varied between fourteen and fifty days.

Transmission. MCV has no animal reservoir, infecting only humans. The condition is very contagious and can be spread through direct and indirect contact, through skin-to-skin contact, and through fomites, especially towels.

Treatment. The growth can be removed with surgery or laser or cryotherapy, or the gradual removal of lesions may be achieved by oral or topical therapy. Oral cimetidine has been used as an alternative treatment for small children since they may not be cooperative either with a surgical removal or the application of topical therapy. Facial mollusca, as well as lesions elsewhere on the body, do not respond to cimetidine.

Podophyllotoxin cream (0.5%) is reliable as a home therapy for men but is not recommended for pregnant women because of its potential toxicity to the fetus. It is more difficult to treat immunocompromised patients, especially patients with HIV/AIDS, because often they do not respond to traditional treatment. Low CD4 cell counts have been linked to widespread facial mollusca and, therefore, have become a marker for a severe HIV disease.

Epidemiology. The disease occurs throughout the world, in both sporadic and epidemic forms, and is more frequent in children than in adults.

Prevention. The best prevention is to follow good hygiene habits. It is important not to touch, pick, or scratch skin that has bumps or blisters. Areas of the body infected with MCV should be kept clean and covered with clothing or a bandage so that others do not touch the bumps and become infected with it. Individuals with molluscum should not take part in contact sports unless all lesions can be covered by clothing or bandages.

Cultures. MCV is cytopathic (cytopathogenic) for human and monkey cell cultures. Virus particles in extracts from lesions of molluscum contagiosum interfere with the growth of other viruses in cultures of mouse embryo cells. However, MCV does not complete the replication cycle in cell culture, and reported growth in cultured human cells has been hard to reproduce.

Family Hepadnaviridae

Hepadnaviruses share with retroviruses the property of encoding reverse transcriptase and replicating via an RNA-to-DNA step, however, somewhat differently. Moreover, they package DNA in the virion and are not particularly closely related to the retroviruses. Hepadnaviridae include three viruses of mammals—hepatitis B virus of primates (HBV), woodchuck hepatitis virus (WHV), and ground squirrel hepatitis virus (GSHV)—and two viruses of birds. The bird viruses form a distinct lineage.

Hepatitis B

Hepatitis B is an acute infection of the liver caused by the hepatitis B virus. Originally, hepatitis B was known as serum hepatitis. Other names that had been used throughout history are yellow fever–vaccine hepatitis, long-incubation hepatitis, homologous serum hepatitis, and posttransfusion hepatitis.

Table 2.8
Properties of Hepatitis B Virus

Alternative name: serum hepatitis

Envelope: from a cell membrane

Capsid: icosahedral

Genome: 3.2 kb, partially ds, circular DNA; one end of the full-length strand is linked to the viral DNA polymerase

Target cell type: hepatocytes

Transmission: sexual intercourse, parenterally, shared contaminated needles, transfusion

Diseases: hepatitis B

Complications: primary hepatocellular carcinoma, cirrhosis (1%–2% mortality)

Therapy: no effective treatment; however, alpha interferon, adefovir dipivoxil, and lamivudine can be used

Prevention: vaccination

Vaccine: subunit/conjugate

In 1940s, British virologist Frank MacCallum coined the term *hepatitis B*. The hepatitis B virus (HBV) is an etiologic agent for hepatitis B. It is a large virus of the hepadnavirus family. The intact virus, a complete virion, is called the Dane particle in reference to D. Dane, the scientist who first saw it by using the electron microscope. The Dane particle has a spherical form. It has an envelope and an icosahedral capsid studded with protein spikes. In the core of this virus is a unique circular DNA that has both a double-stranded and single-stranded section. This DNA is associated with DNA polymerase enzyme.

Under the electron microscope, there are also separate long filamentous *structures* that can be seen. This is called a hepatitis B surface antigen (HBsAg). It is composed of the envelope and some capsid proteins (see Chalkboard Work 2.7). The presence of this structure indicates that the patient has antibodies against the virus and is immune to HBV. Other particles are called hepatitis B core antigen (HBcAg). This is what had been left (icosahedral capsid, DNA, and DNA polymerase) from the virus after the HBsAg (envelope and some proteins) had been removed. As the name implies, it is also antigenic, although antibodies produced against this are not protective.

During viral growth, when an infection is acute, the water-soluble core component called hepatitis B e-surface antigen (HBeAg) is released. If HBeAg is found, this means that the patient has an active disease and is highly contagious. Pregnant women positive on HBeAg in their blood are more likely—90% transmission rate—to transmit HBV to their babies. The transmission rate from the mothers who have no HBeAg is only 10%.

Infectious cycle. When HBV is delivered to the liver, it attaches itself to the surface of the hepatocytes. After uptakes of the virus by the hepatocytes, it travels to the nucleus. The partly double-stranded DNA in the nucleus is then converted into a fully double-stranded, covalently closed circular form (cccDNA) that serves as the template for transcription of the viral RNA. This also serves as a template for reverse transcription, during which viral DNA is built. After the assembly of viral particles, virions are released from infected cells.

Signs and symptoms. Malaise, loss of appetite, muscle and joint pains, low-grade fever, nausea, vomiting, yellow skin, and dark urine are all signs and symptoms of hepatitis B. Many people with a chronic hepatitis B infection may have none of the symptoms and look healthy even though gradual liver damage occurs. The acute illness goes away in two to three weeks; the liver returns to normal function in about four to six months.

Hepatitis B Virus

(HBV)

Dane particle (42nm):

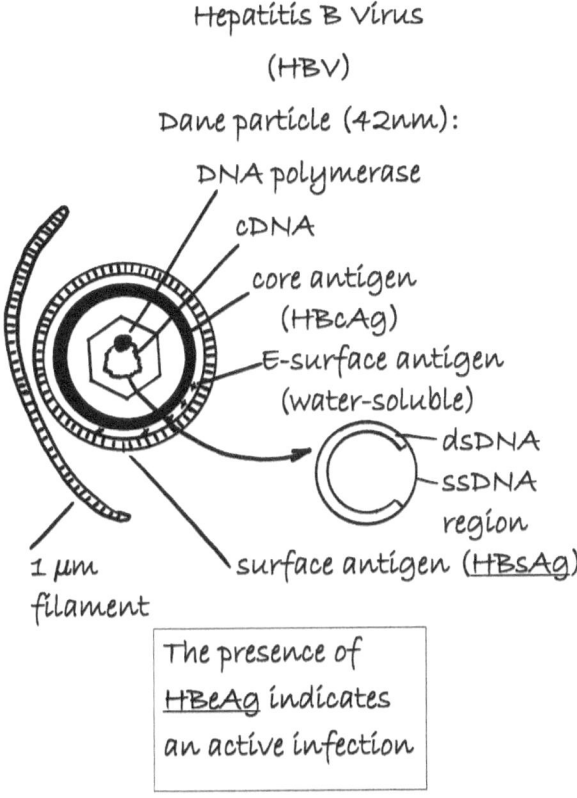

Figure 2.7. Architecture of Hepatitis B virus

Diagnosis. To diagnose hepatitis B, the following tests are generally run:

- HBsAg-positive result indicates an active infection.
- HBcAg-positive result indicates recent infection.
- Antibody to HBsAg (anti-HBc) positive results indicate that patient either had hepatitis B in the past or had been vaccinated.
- HBeAg-positive tests mean the patient is highly contagious.
- A PCR test has been developed to measure the viral load in clinical specimens.

To measure the liver damage done by hepatitis B, the following laboratory work is done:

- Venipuncture to check albumin level
- Liver function tests
- Prothrombin time (PT), a blood test that measures the rate of plasma clotting (normal rate is 11–13.5 seconds)

Incubation period. The incubation period is from seventy to one hundred days.

Sequelae. Cirrhosis is a common complication due to an HBV infection. Fulminant hepatitis leads to liver failure and requires a liver transplant. There is a strong association between HBV membranous glomerulonephritis and hepatocellular carcinoma since HBV causes mutations in host genes that regulate cell growth. The virus also increases susceptibility to exogenous carcinogens.

Transmission. HBV transmission occurs through the exchange of body fluids such as blood, semen, and vaginal secretions (adult horizontal transmission). It is also present in saliva, breast milk, and urine. Without intervention, an HBVinfected mother has a high risk of passing this infection to a child during birth (vertical transmission). Early-life horizontal transmission includes lesions, bites, and sanitary habits. In developing countries, many people still get infected during a blood transfusion due to lack of the resources for proper blood screening.

Hepatitis B is not spread by casual contact such as sharing drinking glasses and eating utensils, holding hands, coughing, sneezing, hugging, or kissing.

Epidemiology. Nearly one-third of the world's population has been infected by HBV. One quarter of a billion people are chronically infected, and therefore, this represents a viral reservoir. Approximately 50% of children born with hepatitis B develop a chronic condition. Only few adults infected with HBV develop chronic hepatitis.

People with chronic hepatitis are considered carriers of the disease even though they do not have symptoms. Worldwide, there are approximately 350 million chronic carriers. High-prevalence areas are China, Southeast Asia, and Africa. Moderate-prevalence areas are Eastern Europe, Russia, and Japan.

Treatment. For a long time, there was no treatment against hepatitis B except regular monitoring of liver function. Now there are alpha interferon, adefovir dipivoxil, and lamivudine treatment. They help only in 35%–40% of cases of hepatitis B. Resting, eating healthy food, drinking plenty of fluids—but no alcohols—are recommended by physicians. Some patients with chronic hepatitis may be treated with antiviral medication (peginterferon). It does not cure but might help to lessen the infection.

Prevention. All children should receive a first dose of hepatitis B vaccine at birth and complete the series of three shots by the sixth to eighteenth month. Health-care workers and those who live with infected individuals should be vaccinated. Immunity against HBV lasts for at least fifteen years. Screening of all who donate blood should be mandatory. The following recommendations should be given to the general public:

- Avoid sexual contact with a person who has acute hepatitis
- Practice safe sex
- Do not share personal items such as razors and a toothbrush
- Do not share needles for drugs, tattooing, or piercing
- Clean blood spills with bleach (one part of household bleach, ten parts of water)

Cultures. HBV cannot be grown on cultured cells.

Historical reference. German scientist Hifiiaryi Lurman made the first record of an epidemic caused by HBV in 1885 in Bremen when 1,289 people were vaccinated against smallpox with lymph from other people; 191 of those vaccinated became jaundiced and were diagnosed with serum hepatitis. Lurman's paper written on this outbreak is now known as a classical study of epidemiology, proving that contaminated lymph were the reason for this outbreak. There had been other outbreaks linked to hepatitis B vaccinations, indicating that the infectious agent was blood-borne. The virus causing the disease was identified in 1965 by an American doctor, Baruch Blumberg.

CHAPTER III

Nonenveloped DNA Viruses

Family Parvoviridae

Parvoviridae is the only family that has a single-stranded DNA as genome and represents the smallest animal DNA viruses. The genome is only about 5 kb in size. Parvovirus virions are nonenveloped and have icosahedral capsid symmetry. Some virions encapsidate the positive strand while others encapsidate the negative. Both nonpathogenic and pathogenic members exist. Parvoviruses infect most vertebrates and many arthropods, causing a variety of diseases.

The family Parvoviridae contains two subfamilies:

- Parvovirinae, which infects vertebrates and include the three genera *Parvovirus*, *Erythrovirus*, and *Dependovirus*
- Densovirinae, which infects invertebrates

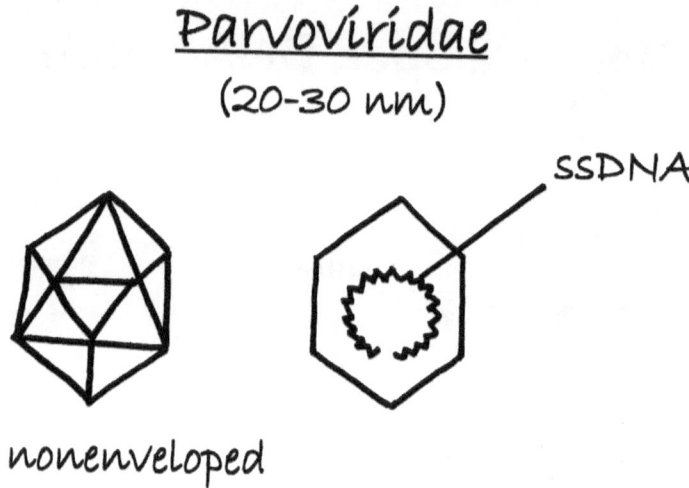

Figure 2.8. Architecture of Parvoviridae

The dependoviruses rely on a helper adenovirus or herpesvirus to supply functions needed for their replication while parvoviruses and erythroviruses do not need a helper virus. Parvovirus B19 is a human pathogen. Most commonly, it causes a mild childhood disease known as erythema infectiosum, but in some cases, it might present more serious symptoms such as aplastic anemia in patients with sickle cell disease, transient arthritis in adults, and more severe anemias due to erythroid marrow failure and rare fetal infections.

Erythema Infectiosum

Table 3.1
Properties of Parvovirus B19

Envelope: none
Capsid: naked, icosahedral
Genome: ssDNA, 5 kb
Target cell type: erythroid progenitor cells
Transmission: droplet contact, direct contact
Diseases: erythema infectiosum (slapped cheek fever, fifth disease)
Diagnosis: ordinarily diagnosed clinically or via EIA, RIA
Symptoms: mild disease with a macular facial rash
Therapy: supportive care
The virus was described by Yvonne Cossart in 1970s.

Erythema infectiosum, also known as a fifth disease, is a common childhood self-limiting disease that causes fever and rash. It is a most common manifestation of parvovirus B19.

Signs and symptoms. The characteristic manifestation is fever with a slapped-cheek appearance with a lacy rash. Within two days, the rash spreads over the body but is most prominent on the arms, legs, and trunk. Other symptoms include fever, itching, and joint pain and swelling.

Diagnosis. Right now, the most sensitive test to detect a recent infection is the IgM antibody assay. Through either enzyme immunoassay (EIA) or radio immunoassay (RIA), antibodies can be detected in about 90% of cases by the third day after the onset of symptoms.

Incubation period. The incubation period for erythema infectiosum is four to twenty-eight days (average sixteen to seventeen days).

Sequelae. Ordinarily, young children recover without any complications while older children may experience mild pruritus (itching), lymphadenopathy, and atypical papular, purpuric, or vesicular rashes. The rash can be exacerbated by sunlight, heat, exercise, and stress for up to three weeks. Immunocompromised people are at risk for serious complications from fifth disease.

Half of all women are immune to fifth disease, and their babies are not at any jeopardy. However, there are some chances that the fetus of those nonimmune women with fifth disease may develop severe anemia, and the woman may have a miscarriage.

Transmission. People with fifth disease are most contagious during the onset of the first symptoms (when it seems like they have "just a cold") before they get the rash or joint pain. The virus is spread into the air in droplets during sneezing and coughing and is passed to a susceptible individual through inhalation since water droplets contain the virus. Unlike with measles, after the rash appears, most of the people are not infectious anymore; people with measles can spread the measles virus when they have the rash.

Treatment. There is no specific treatment for the erythema infectiosum. There are treatments generally for relief of symptoms only. They are usually given to pregnant nonimmune women and immunocompromised individuals.

Epidemiology. Erythema infectiosum occurs worldwide. It can affect any age and can occur sporadically throughout the year. Infection is most common among children of four to ten years of age. By adulthood, 60% of the population is seropositive.

Prevention. Currently, there is no vaccine to prevent infection with B19.

Cultures. In vitro, propagation of parvovirus B19 is primary done in fetal liver culture.

Historical reference. Parvoviruses were discovered in the 1960s. A human pathogen parvovirus B19 was discovered by the virologist Yvonne Cossart in London in the 1970s when she was developing laboratory assays for hepatitis B while working with samples from a hepatitis patient. In fact, the name of the parvovirus B19 was derived from the patient code of one of the viremic blood bank donors. A few years later, the virus was linked with fifth disease, a common rash of childhood.

Family Papovaviridae

Papovaviridae are nonenveloped spherical viruses with icosahedral nucleocapsid. Virions measure 45–70 nm. The genome consists of a single molecule of circularized dsDNA. The virus does not code for any polymerase. The DNA synthesis depends on the host's polymerases. The family is divided into three groups:

- Papillomaviruses
- Polyomaviruses
- Vacuolating viruses

The first group is the most medically important since their members cause warts and cervical cancers. The second group causes tumors in organs of rodents, and the third affects monkeys. Neither polyomaviruses nor vacuolating viruses are associated with human cancer. About 70% of healthy adults are seropositive on polyomaviruses. Preventive procedures are not available and, perhaps, not necessary.

Human Papillomavirus Infections

Table 3.2
Properties of HPV

Envelope: none
Capsid: naked icosahedral (42 capsomers)
Genome: circular, dsDNA, 4–6 kbp
Target cell type: epithelial cells
Transmission: sexual intercourse
Diseases: anogenital warts, cervical cancer, colon cancer, mouth and throat cancer
Treatment: cauterization, regrow after removal
Vaccine: subunit/conjugate

Venereal Warts Infection

A venereal warts infection is a highly infectious, sexually transmitted infection caused by the human papillomaviruses (HPV). HPV subtypes 6, 11, 16, and 18 together are responsible for 70% of cervical cancers and 90% of venereal warts. In addition to warts on genital areas, HPV types 6 and 11 have been associated with conjunctival, nasal, oral, and laryngeal warts. Other names for venereal warts infections are condylomata acuminata, genital warts, anal warts, and anogenital warts.

Signs and symptoms. Incubation period varies from a month to several years. Venereal warts rarely cause discomfort or pain and may look like small flesh-colored bumps and flat lesions, have a cauliflower-like appearance or have tiny stem-like protrusions. In many cases, warts are too small to be seen. In women, venereal warts usually appear on the vulva, on the cervix, or in the vagina. In men, venereal warts usually appear on the scrotum and under the foreskin of an uncircumcised penis and on the shaft of a circumcised penis. In both men and women, a venereal warts infection is associated not only with genital areas of the body but the groin, thighs, and conjunctival, nasal, oral, laryngeal, and anal canal areas. Two strains of HPV contribute to cancers of genitals, anus, mouth, and upper respiratory tract.

Diagnoses. The vinegar solution test can be used to reveal difficult-to-see flat lesions; vinegar turns HPV-infected areas white. A Pap test, also called a Pap smear, is used to collect cervical cells for identification of cancerous or precancerous abnormalities. Lately, doctors are urging anal Pap tests for gay, bisexual men, and straight women who are practicing anal sex and are at higher risk of anal cancer from HPV. The procedure is very simple and may be performed in any doctor's office. The DNA test can recognize the DNA of the high-risk subtypes of HPV that are linked to venereal cancers.

Transmission. The source of the virus is the wart tissue. Transmission occurs by direct or indirect genital skin-to-skin contact with an infected person.

Most often, transmission occurs during penetrative genital contact (oral, vaginal, or anal sex). A person infected with HPV can infect a sex partner even if signs of infection are not apparent. Intra-anal warts are observed predominantly in persons who have had receptive anal intercourse, but they can also occur in men and women who do not have a history of anal sexual contact. Two-thirds of sexual contacts with infected individuals eventually become infected. Using latex condoms does not eliminate the risk of transmitting HPV. A mother with HPV infection may transmit the virus to her infant during delivery. Exposure to the virus may cause infection in the baby's genitals or upper respiratory tract.

Three Groups

3 groups:

Pa = papilloma

= ward

Papillomaviruses

Po = polyoma = tumor

Polyomaviruses

Va = vacuoles = cavities

in infected cells

Vacuolating viruses

Simian virus number 40 (sv40)

Figure 3.1. Classification of Papovaviridae

Epidemiology. Genital HPV infection is the most common sexually transmitted disease in the USA. Approximately 20 million people are currently infected, and 6.2 million Americans become newly infected each year. One study found that more than 42% of urban adolescents had engaged in vaginal intercourse before the age of fourteen, and 40% of them had a sexually transmitted disease. A recent study of girls aged fourteen to nineteen revealed that 18% of them were infected with HPV.

The American Cancer Society estimates about 1,250 men in the USA were diagnosed with cancer of the penis in 2008 and about 2,020 men were diagnosed with anal cancer. The risk of anal cancer is about thirty-five times higher in sexually active gay and bisexual men than in men who have sexual contact only with women. HIV-positive men were estimated to be eighty times more likely to get it.

Treatment. Available therapies for genital warts will likely reduce but probably not eradicate HPV infectivity. Treatment is directed to the macroscopic or precancerous lesions. In many cases, the body's immune system defeats HPV before it has a chance to create any warts. There is no treatment for HPV when no symptoms are present, but there are various ways to treat venereal warts, depending on the size and location. Treatment regiments are classified into patients-applied and provider-applied modalities.

Patient-applied modalities are as follows:

- Podofilox 0.5% solution
- Imiquimod 5% cream
- Sinecatechins (green-tea extract) 15% ointment

Provider-applied modalities are as follows:

- Cryotherapy with liquid nitrogen or cryoprobe
- Podophyllin resin
- Trichloroacetic acid (TCA)
- Bichloroacetic acid (BCA)
- Electrocautery (by electric current)
- Tangential excision: scissor excision, shave excision, or by curettage

No one treatment is better than another. They often come back within a month after treatment. Treating venereal warts will not lower chances of passing HPV to a sex partner. Venereal warts may resolve on their own, stay the same, or grow in size and number. Patients with precancerous and cancerous lesions are referred to a specialist.

Prevention. Two types of vaccine are available: a bivalent Cervarix containing HPV subtypes 16 and 18 and quadrivalent Gardasil containing HPV subtypes 6, 11, 16, and 18. Both vaccines are effective against HPV subtypes that cause cervical, oral, and anal cancers (16 and 18). The quadrivalent is also effective against

HPV subtypes that cause the growth of venereal warts. It has been predicted that immunity of this vaccines will last for five years. However, it is not intended for treatment of those who have already developed cervical, oral, or anal cancer. The vaccine is administrated in three IM injections over a six-month period. The second and third doses should be given two and six months after the first. Missing doses or getting them at the wrong intervals may result in a lower level of immunity or none at all.

The vaccine contains no viral DNA, so there is no threat of developing an HPV infection. It contains no thimerosal or mercury. The most common adverse reactions to Cervarix and Gardasil are local discomfort at the injection site. The vaccines are recommended for both males and females from nine years and older. It is not recommended during pregnancy.

After receiving the vaccine, women still need to continue regular cervical cancer screening with a conventional or liquid-based Pap test because 30% of cervical cancers are caused by HPV subtypes other than 16 or 18. Screening should begin about three years after having vaginal intercourse for the first time.

To prevent the spread of an HPV infection, there should be an increase in the use of Gardasil vaccine in pediatric settings, school clinics, and family settings since the vaccine is two to three times more effective when administrated by age eleven. Adolescents vaccinated when they are young may need boosters later in their lives. Parents should be encouraged to talk openly with their children about responsible sexual behavior and their family's values.

Historical reference. In 2006, the Food and Drug Administration (FDA) in USA approved the human papillomavirus (HPV) vaccine called Gardasil for women. The vaccine had been developed by Merck & Co. In 2009, the vaccine was also approved for men. Currently it is used in the European Union, Australia, the Philippines, Mexico, and Singapore among other countries. Gardasil is a quadrivalent vaccine, which means it works on four HPV subtypes 6, 11, 16, and 18.

Mouth Cancer

According to the National Cancer Institute, oral cancer strikes three hundred thousand Americans each year. Approximately 25% of these cases are fatal due to late detection. There has been a 225% increase in rates of oral cancer from 1974 to 2007. Oral cancer looks like white or red patches in a mouth that bleed easily. As it had been reported at the meeting of the American Association for the Advancement of Science, the primary cause of oral cancer is not smoking or chewing tobacco but human papillomavirus (HPV) contracted through oral sex. This virus is often associated with cervical cancer, but as it turns out, it is not just a health threat for women. More than 60% of the cancers of the mouth and pharynx are caused by HPV. The first scientist to note the link between the virus and oral cancers was Maura Gillison and, as she notes, men and women who had oral sex with six or more partners in their lifetime had an eightfold increase in risk of oral cancer, compared to those who have never performed oral sex.

There is an effective vaccine that had been developed recently. It is called Gardasil and is effective against most common strains of HPV in men and women of any age, not just for women up to twenty-six years of age as had been previously thought. Still, a large number of cases of oral cancer comes from smoking and chewing tobacco, just not as often as had been estimated earlier.

Family Adenoviridae

Table 3.3
Properties of Adenoviridae

Size: 70–90 nm
Envelope: none
Capsid: naked icosahedral (252 capsomers)
Genome: dsDNA, 28–48 kbp (30–40 genes), 5' ends are linked to a terminal protein (TP)

Target cell type: epithelial cells

Transmission: inoculation of conjunctiva (pinkeye), inhalation (acute respiratory infection), fecal-oral route (gastroenteritis)

Reservoir: humans

Diseases: respiratory and gastrointestinal diseases, pharyngoconjunctivitis and keratoconjunctivitis; not purulent

Therapy: supportive care

Vaccine: enteric-coated capsules of the virulent respiratory strains

Administration: oral

Adenovirus was first isolated in the 1950s in adenoid tissue. The Adenoviridae family includes over fifty-two serotypes ubiquitous in human and animal populations. Adenovirus packages a single molecule of double-stranded DNA virus that measures 70–90 nm. The virus has an icosahedral capsid that is formed by the capsomers known as hexons and twelve vertex capsomers known as pentons. From each penton is a fiber projection called fiber antigen. To initiate the reproduction cycle, the virus attaches to the host cell receptor by the fiber antigen. As in all true DNA viruses, transcription of adenovirus's genes depends on the host's polymerases. The virus codes for its own DNA-dependent DNA polymerase.

Upon infection with adenovirus, one of three different interactions with the cells may occur:

- A lytic infection that occurs when an adenovirus enters human epithelial cells and continues through an entire replication cycle, resulting in cytolysis, cytokine production, and the induction of the host inflammatory response.
- A chronic or latent infection that frequently involves an asymptomatic infection of lymphoid tissue.
- Oncogenic transformation has been observed in laboratory rodents.

Members of *Mastadenovirus* genus produce infections of the conjunctiva and respiratory and intestinal tracts. The site of entry generally determines the site of infection; an infection of conjunctiva is due to direct inoculation of the conjunctiva with adenoviruses. Respiratory tract infections result from inhalation of aerosolized droplets while gastrointestinal infections involve a fecal-oral route of transmission. Epidemics of acute keratoconjunctivitis (adenoviral pinkeye) are sometimes associated with visits to eye clinics. Unlike bacterial pinkeye, adenoviral pinkeye is not purulent. The conjunctivae are inflamed with a watery exudate. Adenoviruses are known to cause outbreaks of disease among young military recruits. The infections usually do not require hospitalization and rarely require admission to an ICU. Severe morbidity and mortality associated with adenovirus infections are rare in immunocompetent hosts.

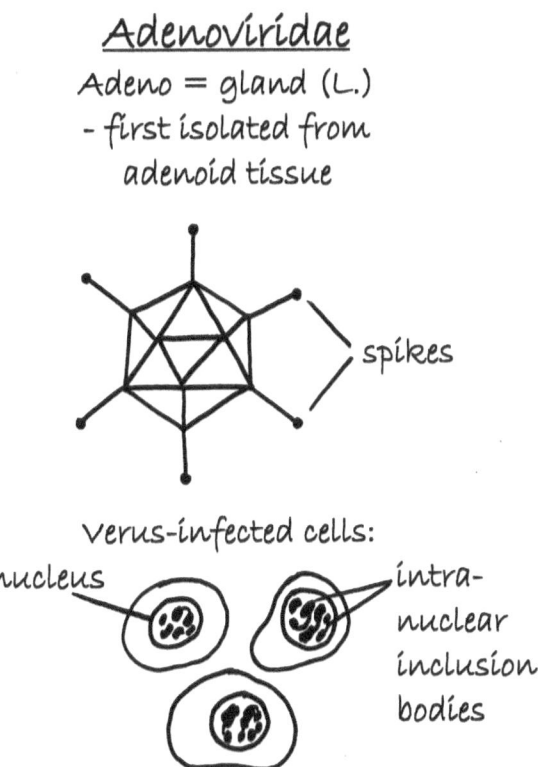

Figure 3.2. Adenoviridae and its inclusion bodies

Most infections are asymptomatic. Uncommon complications that increase the risk of mortality include meningoencephalitis and pneumonia. Mortality rates associated with adenovirus infections among pediatric and adult transplant recipients have varied from 60%–70%.

Adenoviruses survive long periods outside a host and are endemic throughout the year. Vaccines against two serotypes are available, but they are not in general use.

Adenoviruses are cytopathic for human cell cultures, particularly primary kidney and continuous epithelial cells. Growth of the virus in tissue cultures is associated with a stimulation of acid production due to increased glycolysis in the early stages of infection. The cytopathic effect usually consists of a marked rounding and aggregation of affected cells into grapelike clusters. The infected cells do not lyse even though they round up and leave the glass surface on which they have been grown. About seven thousand virus particles are produced per infected cell, and most of them remain intracellular unless means are taken to release them.

CHAPTER IV

Positive Single-Stranded RNA Viruses

Outline

4. West Nile Virus
5. German Measles (Rubella)
VI. Family Coronaviridae
1. Severe Acute Respiratory Syndrome (SARS)
VII. Family Retroviridae

Family Picornaviridae

Mnemonic for picornaviruses is **PEECoRnA**: **P**olio, **E**ntero, **E**cho, **Co**xsackie, **R**hino, and hepatitis **A**.

Picornaviridae comprise one of the largest families of human pathogens. They are very small RNA viruses encompassing nine genera, five of which contain recognized human pathogens. All picornaviruses are closely related. They share significant nucleotide and amino acid sequence identity. The most important are enteroviruses (infecting primarily the enteric tract) and rhinoviruses (infecting primarily the nose and the throat). Over sixty enteroviruses are identified. They replicate primarily in the enteric tract, producing mild diseases. In the heart and CNS, those viruses cause severe symptoms. The enteroviruses are subdivided into polioviruses, Coxsackie viruses, and echoviruses.

The transmission ordinarily occurs through the ingestion of contaminated food or water or direct contact with an individual who excretes the virus. The enteroviruses are resistant to the acid, proteolytic enzymes, and bile of the intestinal contents and may survive for long periods in sewage or even in chlorinated water. They are present in oropharyngeal secretions early after infection and are excreted in feces over a period of weeks following infection. They have the ability to persist in the external environment for weeks.

They have been found in sewages, lakes, and swimming pools. The enteroviruses of nonhuman primates, pigs, cattle, and insects are also known.

Unlike enteroviruses, the rhinoviruses are acid labile but relatively more stable to heat, ordinarily affecting people in the summer and fall. However, they prefer to replicate at 33°C, affecting cooler regions of the respiratory tract, such as nasal passages. They are the causative agents of about half of human colds, frequently causing rhinitis, an inflammation of the nasal mucous membrane, causing a runny nose.

Over a hundred serotypes are identified according to their surface proteins. Children who had not been exposed to rhinoviruses and other viruses that cause colds contract and suffer many cold symptoms each year. Ordinarily, adults become immune to many of the viruses through experience of various cold infections. Rhinoviruses enter via the upper respiratory tract, replicate there, and transmit by direct contact. Coughs and sneezes help spread the viruses to nearby contacts. Histopathologic changes are limited to the mucous membranes: engorgement of blood vessels, edema, mild cellular infiltration, and desquamation of surface cells. These viruses have a limited host range, which has made it necessary to perform all animal experiments in man or in chimpanzees. They have been propagated in cultures of human embryonic lung, diploid human fibroblast tissue, human aortic tissue, and organ cultures of ferret and human tracheal epithelium.

Hepatitis A virus is a picornavirus. Only one serotype is known. It shares only a 28% amino acid identity in its structural proteins with any other picornaviruses, whereas most picornaviruses are more closely related.

Poliomyelitis

Poliomyelitis is an acute infectious disease with poliovirus that in its severest form affects the brain, spinal cord, and certain nerves. The disease is typically characterized by the death of motor neurons in the spinal cord. There are three poliovirus serotypes:

- P1 (Brünhilde)
- P2 (Lansing)
- P3 (Leon)

Table 4.1
Properties of Poliovirus

Size: ~28 nm

Envelope: none

Capsid: icosahedral (32 capsomers)

Genome: +ssRNA, 7–8.5 kb

Reservoir: humans

Target cell type: M cells (?), monocytes (?), macrophages (?), neurons

Transmission: fecal-oral route

Diseases: poliomyelitis

Complications: paralytic disease involving the cranial and respiratory nerves

Therapy: supportive care

Vaccine: inactivated virus (Salk vaccine), attenuated virus (Sabin vaccine)

There is minimal heterotypic immunity between the three serotypes, which means an infection with one serotype does not produce significant immunity to the other serotypes. The poliovirus enters through the mouth. The primary multiplication of the virus occurs at the site of implantation in the pharynx and gastrointestinal tract. Then the virus invades local lymphoid tissue and enters the bloodstream. It may reach the cells of the central nervous system, such as the motor neurons of the anterior horn and the brain stem, where it continues to replicate, causing cell destruction.

Signs and symptoms. Before the onset of symptoms in an infected person, poliovirus is found in the secretions from the mouth and throat and in the feces. Poliomyelitis occurs in four forms:

- Silent or asymptomatic infections, up to 95% of all polio infections, are unapparent. Infected persons without symptoms shed the virus in the stool and are able to transmit the virus to others.
- Abortive infection (4%–8%) results in a minor, nonspecific febrile illness in which cells of the pharynx and the gut are infected. The patient has only the minor illness, characterized by fever, malaise, drowsiness, headache, nausea, vomiting, constipation, or a sore throat in various combinations. There is no clinical or laboratory evidence of a CNS invasion in this form of poliomyelitis.
- Nonparalytic aseptic meningitis (1%–2%) usually follows several days after a prodrome similar to that of a minor illness. The symptoms include stiffness of the neck, back, and/or legs. Ordinarily these symptoms last for two to ten days, followed by a rapid and complete recovery. Poliovirus is only one of many viruses that produce aseptic meningitis.
- Paralytic infection (1%) is the major illness that usually follows the minor illness described above, but it may occur without the antecedent first phase. The predominating complaint is flaccid paralysis resulting from lower motor neuron damage. An incoordination secondary to brain stem invasion and painful spasms of nonparalyzed muscles may also occur. Muscle involvement is ordinarily maximal within a few days after the paralytic phase begins. The maximal recovery generally occurs within six months, but it may take longer.

Diagnosis. Poliovirus may be recovered from the stool or pharynx of a person with poliomyelitis. Isolation of the virus from the cerebrospinal fluid (CSF) is diagnostic but is rarely accomplished.

The CSF usually contains an increased number of white blood cells (10–200 cells/mm^3, primarily lymphocytes) and a slightly elevated protein (40–50 mg/100 mL).

Incubation period. The incubation period ranges from three to thirty-five days.

Sequelae. Some people who survived poliomyelitis develop postpolio syndrome (PPS) years later from which there is no prevention or cure. The symptoms include the following:

- Tiredness
- Muscle weakness
- Joint pain

Transmission. Poliomyelitis is transmitted ordinarily by persons with asymptomatic infections. Individuals infected with poliovirus are most infectious from seven to ten days before and after the onset of symptoms. However, poliovirus may be present in the stool of the infected person from three to six weeks. In addition to airborne transmission, it could be passed through contaminated food and water and multiplied in the intestine, from where it can invade the nervous system.

Treatment. Unfortunately, there is no treatment for polio that can destroy the poliovirus. Therefore, there are only supportive treatments to control the severity of symptoms while the infection runs its course, and they may include the following:

- Rest
- Breathing assistance with a mechanical ventilator
- Acetaminophen or ibuprofen for control of body temperature
- Antibiotics for urinary tract infections
- Bethanechol for urinary retention
- Heating pads and warm towels to reduce muscle pain and spasms

- Painkillers to reduce headache, muscle pain, and spasms (narcotics should not be used due to their effect on breathing)
- Physical therapy for rehabilitation of patients (for instance, braces or corrective shoes could be used to help recover muscle function)

Epidemiology. No reservoir of the infection has been demonstrated in animals. A polio eradication program conducted by the Pan American Health Organization led to elimination of polio in the Western Hemisphere in 1991. Because of the Global Polio Eradication Program, cases of polio had dropped by 99% globally. But later on, the program was thwarted, unable to vaccinate all children and eliminate the last 1% of cases. In an interview for *Science* magazine, CDC's Frieden explained that "for too many people, polio eradication had become a lifestyle rather than a mission." However, in some poorest, marginalized places, it is just impossible to get to, and many vaccinators do not get paid. Polio workers are killed and get death threats in Afghanistan and Nigeria. Another difficulty is mobile populations in Pakistan traveling in and out of the tribal areas where virus circulation is unchecked. Special arrangements have to be made to vaccinate this group of people.

In 2009, 1,579 confirmed cases of polio were reported globally. Poliomyelitis used to occur sporadically or tended to be epidemic. India became the latest country to become polio-free in 2012 after going a full year without registering a new case. However, poliomyelitis remains endemic in three countries: Pakistan, Afghanistan, and Nigeria.

Prevention. Polio can only be prevented by immunization. Inactivated poliovirus vaccine is currently licensed in the United States, but only one vaccine (IPOL, produced by Sanofi Pasteur, SA) is actually distributed. This vaccine contains all three serotypes of the polio vaccine virus. Viruses are grown in a type of monkey kidney tissue culture (Vero cell line) and inactivated with formaldehyde. As a preservative, it contains a mixture of

1. 2-phenoxyethanol,
2. trace amounts of neomycin,
3. trace amounts of streptomycin, and
4. trace amounts of polymyxin B.

The vaccine is administrated through either subcutaneous or intramuscular injection.

Cultures. Poliovirus may be grown in monkeys and chimpanzees. Tissue growth of monkey kidney sustains a generous growth as do certain human cell cultures. The complete replication cycle of poliovirus occurs in an extract of uninfected HeLa cells. The RNA from poliovirus virions, added to such an extract, direct the synthesis of all the poliovirus proteins, replicate RNA, and encapsulate the progeny genomes.

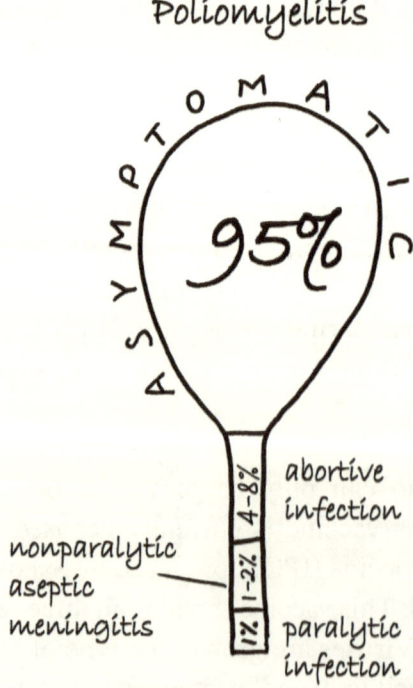

Figure 4.1. Poliomyelitis infections.

Historical. Polioviruses have been important pathogens of humans for a long time. The poliovirus infections were present in ancient Greek and Roman writings. Despite the fact that poliovirus has been widespread in humans for thousands of years, there is no firm evidence of widespread human poliomyelitis until about two hundred years ago. Not until English physician Michael Underwood in 1789 first described debility of the lower extremities in children was poliomyelitis recognizable in England. The poliomyelitis epidemics of large proportions evolved only during the twentieth century. They were concentrated at first in countries practicing the highest standards of hygiene. In the United States, there were huge poliovirus epidemics every summer. By the 1950s, more than five hundred thousand American children and adolescents became ill—twenty thousand of the cases were paralytic, and two thousand to three thousand died. Death was a result of respiratory muscle paralysis. Wards with dozens of patients in iron lungs, first respirators, were a common sight in those epidemics. The machine, called an iron lung, had been invented by Harvard medical researchers Philip Drinker and Louis Agassiz Shaw in 1927. Almost the length of a subcompact car, the iron lung exerted a push-pull motion on the chest.

One of the most known cases of poliomyelitis is that of President Franklin D. Roosevelt, who contracted poliovirus in 1921 at the age of thirty-nine. He was in a wheelchair for the rest of his life. In 1931, the Australians Frank M. Burnet and Jean Macnamara identified the antigenic differences between strains of poliovirus. In 1939, by the persistent efforts of Charles Armstrong, the Lansing strain of poliovirus was adapted to mice, making it available for research purposes in an animal far less expensive than the monkey.

The introduction of the Salk and Sabin vaccines in the 1950s and 1960s led to the elimination of poliovirus in the United States and throughout America. In 1957, just less than six thousand cases of poliomyelitis were reported to the US Public Health Service, of which two thousand five hundred were paralytic. In 1967, there were forty-four cases with twenty-nine paralytic, mostly in unimmunized or inadequately immunized children. Trivalent oral poliovirus vaccine (OPV) was the vaccine of choice in the United States and most other countries after its introduction in 1963. An enhanced-potency inactivated poliovirus vaccine (IPV) became available in 1988. The use of OPV was discontinued in the United States by 2000.

Coxsackie Virus Infections

Table 4.2
Properties of Coxsackie Viruses

Size: ~28 nm
Envelope: none
Capsid: icosahedral
Genome: +ssRNA, 7–8 kb
Target cell type: epithelia
Transmission: respiratory secretions, fecal-oral route
Diseases: A group—hand-foot-mouth disease, herpangina, acute hemorrhagic conjunctivitis, mild not permanent form of paralysis;
B group—pleurodynia
Both A and B groups: febrile upper respiratory infections (rhinitis, pharyngitis), orchitis, aseptic (viral) meningitis, meningoencephalitis, and myopericarditis
Therapy: supportive care

Coxsackie virus infections are common eye and upper respiratory infections and less common infections of the heart and CNS. Coxsackie viruses cause infections in both adults and children; the severity of the infections varies from mild to life-threatening. Coxsackie viruses are divided into two groups. This classification is based on early observations of their pathogenicity in laboratory mice. Group A coxsackie viruses cause muscle injury, paralysis, and death in mice; group B causes less severe outcomes but results in mice organ damage. Each group is divided into over twenty-four serotypes distinguished by different proteins on their surfaces.

The virus is resistant to stomach acid and can survive outside the body on surfaces for hours. The situation, as far as distribution of viruses is concerned, is similar to that found in poliomyelitis.

Signs and symptoms. These viruses cause a large variety of symptoms.

1. The A group of coxsackie viruses causes the following:
    *   A generalized rash or clusters of red spots that may appear in some coxsackie infections. It may cause blisters on the palms and soles of the feet and inside the mouth (tongue, gums, and cheeks) along with a fever and a sore throat. This condition is known as hand-foot-mouth disease (HFMD); usually, vesicles are not pruritic, which helps to distinguish this condition from chicken pox. Herpangina is common in children of three to ten years of age during the summer months and characterized by fever, sore throat, and tender blisters in the mouth but not on the palms or soles of the feet.
    *   Acute hemorrhagic conjunctivitis (AHC) manifests with a swollen eye and red hemorrhages in the whites of the eye. The infection usually spreads to the other eye. Symptoms usually resolve in a week or so.
    *   Weakness in an arm or leg, sometimes with partial paralysis. This uncommon symptom resembles poliomyelitis but in mild form, and the paralysis is not permanent.

2. The B group of coxsackie viruses causes the following:
    *   Pleurodynia or Bornholm disease is an inflammation of the muscles in the chest that feels like a sharp chest pain especially when person takes a deep breath. This pain comes and goes in waves. The infection might resolve on its own in about five days or persist for a few weeks.

3. Both A and B groups of coxsackie viruses can cause the following:
   • Febrile upper respiratory infections with a sore throat and a runny nose. In some people it causes a cough somewhat similar to bronchitis. However, it is rare when coxsackie viruses cause pneumonia.
   • Aseptic (viral) meningitis—during the disease, children become lethargic and febrile seizures may occur. Adults complain of headache, fever, and neck stiffness. In some cases, a rash may appear.
   • Meningoencephalitis usually occurs in small children; this severe condition occurs infrequently.
   • Myopericarditis, an inflammation of the heart and lining of the heart. This manifestation of coxsackie viruses is extremely rare. It could be mild or severe, causing a heart attack and death. The injuries to the heart may be transient or permanent. The condition manifests with shortness of breath, chest pain, fatigue, and leg swelling. Children with myopericarditis usually fare better than adults.

Coxsackie virus may cause syndrome similar to infectious mononucleosis. In young boys, coxsackie viruses may cause orchitis, a testicle infection. Infants, rather than older children, are at a higher risk to get severe illness, such as myopericarditis, hepatitis, pneumonia, and life-threatening diarrhea diseases that may be fatal.

Incubation period. The incubation period for coxsackie viruses is highly variable and in the range of two to thirty-five days, the most common being three to six days.

Sequelae. Mortality due to a Coxsackie virus infection is uncommon, though these viruses appear to be a danger in early and late stages of pregnancy.

Diagnoses. Patients with symptoms of a common cold or a rash usually do not require any laboratory tests. Patients with conjunctivitis are examined by using an ophthalmoscope to confirm the diagnosis. A slit lamp examination may reveal keratitis. A swab from patients with a sore throat is taken to rule out strep throat.

Physician may require a spinal tap since many patients show an increased number of leucocytes in the cerebrospinal fluid, a normal sugar level, and a slight increase in the protein level. The PCR can detect 65%–90% of infections.

Myopericarditis requires evaluation with an electrocardiogram (ECG or EKG) to evaluate rhythms of the heart and to indicate whether or not the sac of the heart is inflamed. An echocardiogram, an ultrasound of the heart, evaluates the size of the heart, how well it pumps blood, and whether or not there is a fluid around the heart.

Transmission. The virus is spread from person to person through respiratory secretions and bodily fluids. It may also be cast off in the stool, making a fecal-oral route of transmission. People are most contagious during the first week of illness, but the virus may be present during a period of convalescence as well. The weaker the immune system, the longer the virus exists in the body.

Epidemiology. Viruses of the coxsackie group have been encountered around the globe. Infections occur at all ages, although it is more common in infants and children. It is more common in males, with a male-to-female ratio of 2:1. About ten million symptomatic enteroviral infections occur in the USA annually; coxsackie viruses accounted for 24% of those infections. In 2007, there was an outbreak of Coxsackie virus infection in China, resulting in two hundred children hospitalized and twenty-two childhood deaths. More than eight hundred people were affected.

Treatment. There are no drugs that destroy the virus. Fortunately, coxsackie infections resolve on their own, as soon as two days or up to two weeks. Acetaminophen and ibuprofen can be used to reduce pain and fever. The use of aspirin should be avoided because of the risk of Reye's syndrome. In severe cases, hospitalization is required for supportive therapy.

Prevention. To prevent infection, hands should be washed frequently by both sick and well people, and one should cover one's mouth when coughing or sneezing. Contaminated surfaces should be cleaned with household bleach (1 teaspoon of bleach to 4 cups of water). People who feel ill should stay home to prevent infection from spreading. There is no vaccine against coxsackie viruses.

Cultures. The virus growth in the laboratory either multiplies in the tissue cultures or in suckling mice.

Historical reference. The Coxsackie virus was discovered by Gilbert Dalldorf in 1948–1949 in the USA. He was searching for the cure for polio while collaborating with Grace Sickles. Working with experimental mice, he discovered the viruses that mimic mild nonparalytic polio. The virus was named after the small town in New York—Coxsackie, where Dalldorf obtained the first fecal specimens.

Hepatitis A

Hepatitis A is an acute infection of the liver caused by the hepatitis A virus (HAV). In different countries, hepatitis A (HAP) used to have different names. In Russia, it had been called "Botkin's disease"; in England, "infectious hepatitis"; in France, "jaunisse des camps"; in India and Pakistan, "urgan" or "palia"; in the USA, catarrhal jaundice, epidemic hepatitis, and short-incubation hepatitis. In 1940, a British doctor, F. O. MacCallum, proposed to use the term *viral hepatitis type A*.

Table 4.3
Properties of Hepatitis A Virus

Alternative name: infectious hepatitis

Size: ~28 nm

Envelope: none

Capsid: icosahedral capsid

Genome: +ssRNA, 7–8.5 kb

Target cell type: hepatocytes

Transmission: fecal-oral, often food-borne

Diseases: hepatitis A, no chronic infections; no association with cancer

Complications: serious liver damage, liver failure

Therapy: supportive care

Vaccine: inactivated virus

The etiologic agent is a nonenveloped, positive-stranded virus RNA of the Picornaviridae family. There are many genotypes of the virus but only one serotype. After being ingested by humans, HAV reaches the intestine, where it is absorbed into the bloodstream and delivered to the liver through the portal system. In the liver, it starts replicating, shedding in high concentration in feces.

Signs and symptoms. In patients with hepatitis, the skin or the eyes become jaundiced. Other signs and symptoms may include severe abdominal pain, gray-colored stools, vomiting, fever, joint pain, malaise, and a loss of appetite. Symptoms are more severe in adults than in children, although some adults and many children have no such symptoms.

Diagnosis. Diagnosis is done by blood samples. Serology tests might reveal raised titer of IgM and IgG antibodies and elevated liver enzymes.

Incubation period. First symptoms appear between fifteen and forty-five days after the initial infection.

Sequelae. Death is rare, about 3–5 in 1,000 adults under fifty, and 18 in 1,000 elderly individuals.

Transmission. HAV is most commonly spread from person to person through fecally contaminated water or food or by oral-anal contact with an infected person. A parenteral route of transmission is possible but very rare.

Epidemiology. Tens of millions of people throughout the world become infected every year. It has been estimated that 40% of acute viral hepatitis is caused by HAV. In 1988, 300,000 people in Shanghai were infected with HAV by eating clams from contaminated water. In 2003, there was an outbreak in Ohio when about 640 people were infected, four of whom died. The outbreak was linked to green onions served at a single restaurant. To date, 20,000 people in the USA become infected with HAV annually. Because of vaccination, there was 90% reduction in HAV cases in the USA.

Treatment. Hepatitis A is a self-limiting disease that does not cause chronic liver infection or chronic liver disease. There is no treatment for hepatitis A other than resting, excluding alcohol and fatty foods from the diet, staying hydrated, and eating well-balanced meals. Analgesics are used to reduce abdominal pain; antiemetics are used to avoid nausea and vomiting.

Prevention. Inactivated hepatitis A vaccine protects against infection for longer than twenty years and is recommended for all one-year-old children as well as health-care professionals and travelers to countries where personal hygiene and sanitary conditions are poor in Central and South America, Asia (except Japan), Africa, and Eastern Europe. In the environment, HAV can be inactivated by chlorine treatment, formalin, beta-Propiolactone, and UV radiation.

Cultures. HAV grow in cultures of liver cells of such primates as marmosets. The virus is resistant to detergents, acid (pH 1), solvents (chloroform, ether), and drying and survives temperatures under 60°C. It can be inactivated by boiling for five minutes. Moreover, it can survive for months in fresh and salted water.

Family Flaviviridae

The Flaviviridae are divided into three genera:

- The *Flavivirus* genus, members of which cause yellow fever, dengue fever, Japanese encephalitis, and such tick-borne encephalitides as Central European encephalitis (CEE), louping ill, Russian spring-summer encephalitis (RSSE), Kyasanur Forest disease, Omsk hemorrhagic fever, and Powassan encephalitis.
- The *Pestivirus* genus, members of which cause bovine diarrhea and classical swine fever virus.
- The *Hepacivirus* genus, members of which cause hepatitis C in humans.

The flavivirus genome is ~11–12 kb, which is comprised of a positive-sense, single-stranded RNA molecule. The flavivirus virion is ~50 nm in diameter and is comprised of an electron-dense nucleocapsid core surrounded by an endoplasmic reticulum-derived lipid bilayer. Certain viruses belonging to the family Flaviviridae have long been known to be competent to undergo recombination.

Flaviviridae
(flavus = yellow)

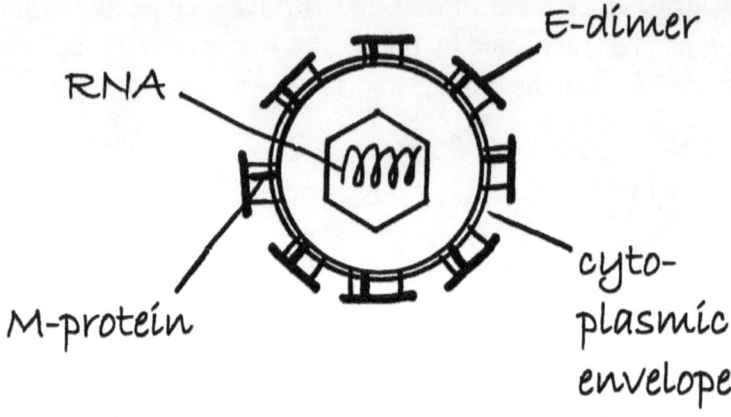

Figure 4.2. Architecture of Flaviviridae

Hepatitis C

In addition to rock 'n' roll, drugs, sexual liberation, and shaggy hair, baby boomers can also lay claim to the hepatitis C virus (HCV) as a defining feature of their generation.

—Jon Cohen, *Science*, 2012

Hepatitis C is an acute infection of the liver caused by the hepatitis C virus (HCV). Alternative names are non-A hepatitis, non-B hepatitis, or chronic hepatitis. HCV is a virus of the *Hepacivirus* genus, the Flaviviridae family.

Table 4.4
Properties of Hepatitis C Virus

Alternative name: posttransfusion hepatitis

Virion: spherical, ~30–60 nm

Envelope: from cytoplasmic membrane

Capsid: icosahedral

Genome: +ssRNA, ~11–12 kb

Target cell type: hepatocytes

Transmission: parenteral and sexual transmission; sharing toothbrush, razor blade, a straw to snort drugs, or needles while injecting drugs

Diseases: hepatitis C, an acute and usually subclinical; it has high rate of chronicity, with 1%–2% mortality

Vaccine: none

Signs and symptoms. Most people who have been infected with HCV have no symptoms until the onset of chronic hepatitis and cirrhosis occurs; the progression of the disease is indolent. Symptoms are mild, nonspecific, and include fatigue, abdominal pain, dark urine, jaundice, loss of appetite, low-grade fever, nausea, and vomiting. Sometimes, it takes twenty to forty years to reach its end point.

Diagnosis. At this time, there is no test that distinguishes between those who are infectious and those who are fully recovered and no longer infectious. Diagnoses include the following tests:

- An ELISA
- A hepatitis C genotype analysis
- A RNA assay to detect a viral load

To determine liver damage, the same tests are run as with patients with hepatitis B. A liver biopsy might also be requested.

Incubation period. The incubation period is from forty-two to forty-nine days. However, 60%–70% of infected people do not have any symptoms and, therefore, are unaware of the infection.

Sequelae. The silent onset of hepatitis C symptoms eventually leads to chronic hepatitis and cirrhosis. It is the leading cause of liver cancer in the USA. HCV causes cirrhosis in about 20% of people infected for longer than twenty years.

Transmission. Since transmission occurs primarily through blood exchange, risk groups include people who use illegal drugs by sharing needles, patients who had a blood transfusion before July 1992, people who received blood clotting factors concentrates before 1987, persons who were on long-term dialysis, health-care professionals who have had mucosal exposure to HCV-positive blood, individuals who have multiple sex partners, and children born to HCV-positive mothers.

The risk of passing hepatitis C from a pregnant woman to her baby is low; the transmission rate is only 5%. The virus is transmitted through birth, and there is no way to reduce the risk. As with hepatitis B, there is no evidence that hepatitis C can be transmitted through casual contact. It could not be passed through breast-feeding unless the nipple is bleeding. However, the virus can live outside the body for a week and, thus, can cause infection by sharing a toothbrush, a razor blade, or a straw to snort drugs.

Epidemiology. An estimate of 270–300 million people are infected with hepatitis C worldwide, about 4 million in the USA. It is estimated that 40%–60% of all chronic liver diseases in the USA are due to hepatitis C. Males are twice as likely to be infected as females. Recent studies show that HCV prevalence among prison inmates is three to five times greater than in the general population.

To date, the highest rate of HCV infection in the world is in Egypt; half a million Egyptians are infected with the diseases each year. Most infections stem from unsterilized, used needles to inject villagers with treatments for the chronic illness of schistosomiasis, a parasitic infection.

Treatment. New drugs, simeprevir (Olysio) and sofosbuvir (Sovaldi) for HCV are now available in the United States. The cost of these drugs ranges from $66,000 to $84,000 per person, for a 12-week course of treatment. Newer drugs, daclatasvir and 3D, are undergoing regulatory review. Thus, To date, there is no affordable cure for the patients. More than half of those who get hepatitis C never fully recover when old drugs are used. Often, interferon alfa, which has serious side effects, and Ribavin are prescribed for treatment. However, synthetic interferons become rapidly broken down by the body within twelve to twenty-four hours. After this distraction, there are no interferons left to suppress or destroy HCV.

Prevention. There are no vaccines against hepatitis C. Preventing the spread of the infection includes identifying people at risk, HCV testing, changing the behavior that puts people at risk of a HCV infection, the use of latex condoms to prevent body fluid exchange, the reduction of the number of the sex partners, continuing medical education programs, and increasing public awareness through advertisements. It is crucial that people who learn their status receive proper medical care.

Cultures. Usually, HCV cannot be grown in cultured cells. The only susceptible laboratory animal is the chimpanzee. In 2005, scientists at the National Institute of Diabetes and Digestive and Kidney Diseases (NIDDK) were able to replicate the HCV in a test tube.

Historical reference. While tested negative for hepatitis A and B, many patients in the 1970s still developed an acute form of hepatitis. At that time, scientists called it non-A and non-B hepatitis; we now suspect that 90%–95% of these cases were actually hepatitis C, not acknowledged until 1988, when the causative agent, HCV, had been identified. During the 1980s, HCV infected 230,000 Americans each year. After a blood test for hepatitis C had been perfected in 1992, it eliminated HCV from the blood transfusion supply, reducing the chance of anyone coming down with hepatitis C through a blood transfusion to 0.01%.

It is not known for how long hepatitis C had been around since blood samples from different periods of time are not available. It is difficult to trace the origin of hepatitis C since the virus causing it had been found in remote areas all over the world.

Hepatitis G

Table 4.5
Properties of Hepatitis G Virus

Virion: spherical, ~50 nm
Envelope: from cytoplasmic membrane
Capsid: icosahedral
Genome: +ssRNA, ~11–12 kb
Target cell type: hepatocytes
Transmission: blood-borne, sexual transmission
Diseases: hepatitis G
Vaccine: none

Hepatitis G is an infection caused by hepatitis G virus (HGV). HGV is an often used anachronism to the GB virus (GBV) infection, named after the surgeon G. Barker, who fell ill in 1966 with a non-A, non-B hepatitis.

Causative agent. GBV belongs to the family of Flaviviridae, but it is not assigned to any of its genus. GBV role in hepatitis has not been confirmed. It replicates primarily in lymphocytes and poorly on hepatocytes.

Signs and symptoms. GBV infections are usually mild and brief.

Diagnosis. The only method used to detect GBV is a very costly DNA test.

Incubation period. Incubation period is unknown.

Sequelae. There is no evidence that hepatitis G can cause serious complications. Many researchers doubt that HGV is capable of causing any disease. Some studies suggest that its coinfection with HGV actually slows the HIV disease.

Transmission. Hepatitis G is a blood-borne infection. People who require a large amount of blood or blood products, patients who have a kidney disease that require hemodialysis, and intravenous drug users are at risk of hepatitis G. Mothers might pass it to the newborns, and there also might be a possibility of sexual transmission.

Treatment. There is no specific treatment of any kind for hepatitis G. Patients are recommended to use a balanced diet, avoid alcohol, and rest in bed.

Epidemiology. HGV has been identified in as many as 20% of patients who have long-lasting viral hepatitis infections, including hepatitis C. An estimate of 2% of US healthy blood donors are viremic with GBV.

Prevention. Since hepatitis G is a blood-borne infection, prevention relies on avoiding contact with contaminated blood.

Cultures. GBV replication is inefficient *in vitro*; therefore, there is no reliable culture system for it.

Historical reference. GBV was first described in 1995.

HGV is similar to HCV; both are Flaviviridae.

Figure 4.3. HGV and HCV

Yellow Fever

Yellow fever is an acute febrile hemorrhagic disease caused by the RNA virus of the Flaviviridae family transmitted to humans either by the yellow fever mosquito (*Aedes aegypti*) or the tiger mosquito (*Aedes albopictus*). Alternative names are jungle yellow fever, urban yellow fever, black vomit, yellow jack, and American plague.

Table 4.6
Properties of Yellow Fever Virus

Virion: spherical, ~50 nm

Envelope: from cytoplasmic membrane

Capsid: icosahedral

Genome: +ssRNA, ~11–12 kb

Target cell type: dendritic cells, Kupffer cells, hepatocytes

Vector: mosquitoes *Aedes aegypti* or *Aedes albopictus*

Reservoir: monkeys

Diseases: yellow fever, hepatitis

Complication: hemorrhagic fever

Vaccine: attenuated virus (for travelers to endemic areas)

The virus enters through the skin and then spreads to the local lymph nodes, where it multiplies. From the lymph nodes, it enters the circulating blood and becomes localized in the liver, spleen, kidney, bone marrow, and lymph glands. Even after the virus has become cleared from the blood, it may still be present for days in the lymph nodes, the spleen, and the bone marrow. The presence and propagation of the virus in a particular organ may lead to a formation of lesions that can cause severe necrosis especially in the liver and the kidney, which eventually results in the host's death.

During the recovery period, the parenchymatous cells are replaced, and the liver may be completely restored. Degenerative changes also occur in the spleen, the lymph nodes, and the heart.

Signs and symptoms. In general, the clinical severity of an illness ranges from a self-limited febrile illness to a severe hepatitis and hemorrhagic fever. Symptoms include chills, high fever, arrhythmias, decreased urination, delirium, myalgias, vomiting, red eyes, red face and tongue, seizures, and coma. A total of 5%–10% of all diagnosed cases are fatal, and 20%–50% of those patients who become jaundiced die of the infection.

Incubation period. The incubation period is three to six days.

Sequelae. Complications of yellow fever include bacterial meningitis, encephalitis, nerve damage, liver failure, necrosis of the kidney or the stomach, myocarditis, excessive bleeding, and pneumonia.

Diagnoses. It is difficult to distinguish yellow fever on the basis of signs and symptoms from other diseases, especially in the early stages of the disease. Laboratory diagnosis is accomplished by testing the serum or the cerebrospinal fluid to detect the virus-specific IgM and neutralizing antibodies.

Transmission. The only known hosts of the yellow fever virus are primates and several species of mosquitoes. Yellow fever is transmitted by the bite of an infected yellow fever mosquito, *Aedes aegypti*, or a tiger mosquito, *Aedes albopictus*. The female mosquito takes up the virus during feeding. The virus then replicates in the mosquito's gut. When the mosquito feeds again, the virus passes through the mosquito's saliva to the next host, causing viremia.

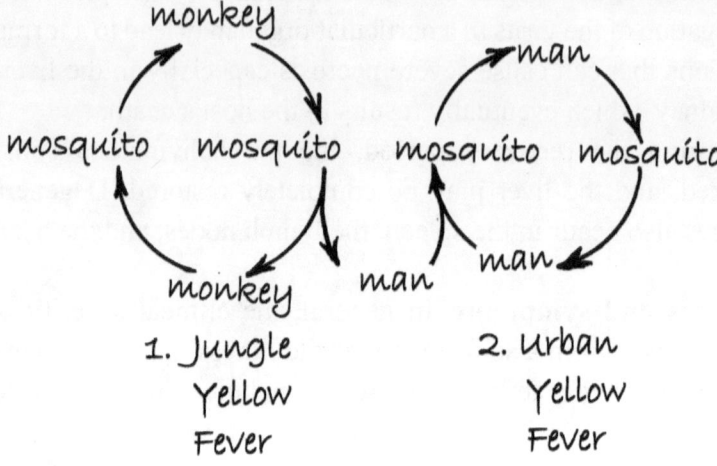

Figure 4.4. Transmission of yellow fever

Epidemiology. Yellow fever occurs in tropical regions of Africa and Central and South America. According to WHO, yellow fever causes two hundred thousand illnesses and thirty thousand deaths every year in unvaccinated populations. Around 90% of cases occur in Africa. The last epidemic of yellow fever in North America occurred in 1905 in New Orleans.

Treatment. There is no treatment to combat the yellow fever virus; therefore, treatment is symptomatic rest, which includes the use of ibuprofen, naproxen, acetaminophen, or paracetamol to relieve symptoms of fever and aching. Dehydration can be treated with fluids through a vein or with oral rehydration solution. Aspirin should be avoided. Patient should have no exposure to the mosquito to prevent the transmission cycle. Most people get better after a long recovery period.

Prevention. Steps to prevent yellow fever include the following:

- Staying in well-screened, air-conditioned areas as much as possible.
- Use of a bed net when sleeping.

- Use of protective clothing such as long-sleeved shirts and long pants; for extra protection, treated clothing with insecticide permethrin.
- Use of insect repellent containing DEET (N,N-diethylmetatoluamide), picaridin (KBR 3023), IR3535, p-Menthane (PMD), or oil of lemon eucalyptus are effective. Instructions on the label have to be carefully followed.
- Vaccination. Vaccine is given as a onetime shot. Yellow fever vaccine contains a strain of an attenuated virus called 17D. For people who are at risk, a booster dose is recommended every ten years. People who are allergic to eggs, chicken protein, or gelatin should not get vaccinated.

Cultures. Yellow fever virus is readily cultivated in the developing chick embryo and in tissue cultures made from chick or mouse embryos. All strains of the virus produce encephalitis in mice following direct inoculation into the brain.

Historical Reference. Epidemics followed the trade ships from Africa to America. In 1937, South African American virologist Max Theiler developed a safe and highly effective vaccine for yellow fever virus for which he received the 1951 Nobel Prize in Physiology and Medicine.

Dengue Fever

Dengue fever is a febrile tropical disease caused by a variety of dengue viruses of the Flaviviridae family and is transmitted by the bite of infected female mosquitoes *Aedes aegypti* or *Aedes albopictus*. This infectious disease is also known as breakbone fever. Infection of monocytes results in release of vasoactive mediators, which cause the increased vascular permeability and hemorrhagic manifestations characterized as dengue hemorrhagic fever or dengue shock syndrome.

Table 4.7

Properties of Dengue Fever Virus

Virion: spherical, ~50 nm

Envelope: from cytoplasmic membrane

Capsid: icosahedral

Genome: +ssRNA, ~11 kb

Target cell type: monocytes, but not T or B cells

Vector: female mosquitoes *Aedes aegypti* or *Aedes albopictus*

Reservoir: mammals

Diseases: Dengue fever

Complications: dengue hemorrhagic shock syndrome

Vaccine: none

Causative agent. Dengue fever is caused by any of four closely related viruses of the following serotypes:

- DENV-1
- DENV-2
- DENV-3
- DENV-4

Following the introduction of the virus by the bite of the mosquito, there is local edema and erythema as a result of local multiplication of the virus. The virus is present in the high serum in the high titer within twenty-four hours after the first rise in temperature. The histopathologic lesion is in and about the capillaries, producing endothelial swelling, perivascular edema, and infiltration with mononuclear cells. A person can be affected only once by the same type of virus.

Signs and symptoms. The severity of an illness ranges from a self-limited febrile illness to a severe dengue hemorrhagic fever (DHF). Symptoms begin with a high fever, a severe headache, a pain behind the eyes, arthralgia, myalgia, bone pain, a rash, tendency to bruise easily, and nose and gum bleeding. A flushed face and injected conjunctivitis are common. DHF is characterized by a fever that lasts for four to seven days; when it declines, symptoms include persistent vomiting, severe abdominal pain, and difficulty breathing. The temperature may raise again, a "saddleback" form. A rash appears on the third or fourth day, and the lymph nodes enlarge. During this stage, capillaries become excessively permeable and, in addition, the platelet count drops low. Consequently, blood fluid escapes into the peritoneum, causing accumulation of fluid (ascites), and into the pleural cavity, causing pleural effusion. Convalescence may take weeks; however, the pathogenic effects may cause failure of the circulatory system, leading to dengue shock syndrome and death.

Most people (80%) with dengue fever are either asymptomatic or have very mild symptoms such as only a fever, but in both cases, they may transmit their infection to mosquitoes. Unlike yellow fever, mortality rates are low.

Incubation period. The time between exposure and the onset of symptoms ranges from four to seven to three to fourteen days. A laboratory worker developed dengue nine days after serum from a patient had been accidently squirted in his eye.

Sequelae. While children often experience symptoms similar to a common cold or gastroenteritis, they are more susceptible to complications such as brain damage, myocarditis, liver failure, dengue shock syndrome, and death.

Diagnoses. Clinically, dengue fever is often misdiagnosed as influenza, measles, typhoid fever, or malaria. Laboratory diagnoses include detection of antidengue IgM and IgG by indirect ELISA. Specific serotypes can be identified by indirect fluorescent antibody testing.

Transmission. Like yellow fever, dengue fever cannot be directly spread from person to person, although there is evidence that dengue fever can be transmitted from mother to fetus. Rarely is dengue fever transmitted through blood transfusion or organ transplant. Usually, the disease is transmitted through the bite of an infected mosquito—either *Aedes aegypti* or *Aedes albopictus*, which have a greater affinity for humans than many other mosquito vectors. After a mosquito's infected blood meal, the virus requires eight to twelve days incubation before it can transmit the infection to humans. The mosquito remains infected for the rest of its life.

Epidemiology. In many tropical and subtropical countries of Southern Asia, Africa, Central and South America, and the Pacific Ocean, dengue fever is endemic. Currently, 40% of the world's population lives in areas where there is a risk of dengue fever infection. Fifty to one hundred million people get infected annually, and five hundred thousand of them develop DHF that causes twenty-two thousand deaths, mostly in children.

Treatment. As with yellow fever, there is no specific treatment for dengue fever. Only supportive therapy can be conducted, which includes bed rest, fluid replacement, and the use of analgesics with acetaminophen; the use of analgesics with aspirin should be avoided.

Prevention. There is no vaccine for dengue fever. Prevention of dengue fever could be achieved by community-based mosquito control. To prevent mosquitoes from laying their eggs, containers that collect or store water should be covered or properly discarded. At least once a week, pet and animal watering containers should be emptied and cleaned after use. Proper application of mosquito repellents containing 20%–30% DEET decreases the risk of being bitten by mosquitoes. Windows and doors should be screened.

Cultures. Dengue virus grows to high levels in cultures of monkey kidney, hamster kidney, and HeLa cells, producing cytopathic changes.

Historical reference. Dengue fever is an emerging disease. Dengue viruses originated in Africa or Southeast Asia between one hundred and eight hundred years ago. It was a geographically restricted disease until the middle of the twentieth century, when the disease was disseminated to about one hundred countries by the coincidental transport of *Aedes* mosquitoes. It was not until 1981 that numerous cases of dengue fever began to appear in the Caribbean and Latin America. The most recent outbreak occurred in Puerto Rico in 2007, when more than ten thousand cases were diagnosed. The high-transmission season begins in August, continuing until November. The Australian Red Cross had to discard 33,600 liters of donated blood for fear it was contaminated with dengue fever after a large Northern Queensland outbreak in 2009–2010.

Family Caliciviridae

Caliciviridae are distant relatives of the Picornaviridae, though, unlike the most of the Picornaviridae, they produce at least one subgenomic RNA. Caliciviridae cause a wide spectrum of diseases in animals, including respiratory infections, vesicular lesions, gastroenteritis, and hemorrhagic disease. They are important etiologic agents of acute gastroenteritis in humans and, therefore, are also referred to as human caliciviruses (HuCVs). The first described calicivirus was a virus of sea lions. The human caliciviruses have been difficult to study.

Table 4.8
Properties of Caliciviridae

Size: ~35–40 nm
Envelope: none
Capsid: naked icosahedral
Genome: +ssRNA, nonsegmented, ~7.5–8.5 kb
Transmission: food-borne (potluck meals, contaminated shellfish), waterborne, inhalation
Diseases: respiratory infections, vesicular lesions; gastrointestinal (noninflammatory diarrhea) and hemorrhagic disease

---

What we know of the molecular biology of this group of viruses comes from studies of nonhuman viruses. Viruses genetically and antigenically closely related to HuCVs have also been isolated from animals. The family Caliciviridae consists of four genera: *Norovirus* (NV), *Sapovirus* (SV), *Lagovirus*, and *Vesivirus*. They are all nonenveloped viruses with icosahedral symmetry and a positive-sense, single-stranded polyadenylated RNA genome.

Family Hepeviridae

Because of similarity in the organization of the genomes at one time, the hepatitis E virus (HEV) was considered a member of Caliciviridae family. Sequence analysis has suggested that HEV should be reclassified. The International Committee on Taxonomy of Viruses has created a new family, Hepeviridae, with HEV as the prototypic member of the genus *Hepevirus*. Hepeviridae are nonenveloped, positive single-stranded RNA viruses that have pronounced spikes on the capsid and are approximately 7,200 nt (nucleotide) in length.

Hepatitis E

Hepatitis E is an acute infection of the liver caused by the hepatitis E virus (HEV). The etiological agent of hepatitis E resembles hepatitis A (HAV). There are at least two strains of HEV—one found in Asia, another in Mexico. The virus might divide in the gastrointestinal tract, but the most common place for its replication is the liver.

Table 4.9
Properties of Hepatitis E Virus

Alternative name: enteric hepatitis
Size: 32–34 nm in diameter
Capsid: naked icosahedral, 60 capsid proteins
Envelope: none

Genome: linear, +ssRNA, three partially overlapping ORFs, 7.2 kb
Transmission: fecal-oral, water, shellfish
Diseases: hepatitis E, no chronic infections, no association with cancer
Complications: 20% mortality in pregnant women
Vaccine: none

Signs and symptoms. Symptoms associated with acute HEV infections may be more severe than those induced by HAV, still clinically indistinguishable from hepatitis A. HEV infection includes the same signs and symptoms such as malaise, loss of appetite, abdominal pain, arthralgia, nausea, dark urine, pale-colored stool, and fever. Infection with hepatitis E is often subclinical. In pregnant women, HEV infection can be life-threatening.

Diagnosis. Hepatitis E can be distinguished only serologically. Epidemiological characteristics have to be taken into consideration as well.

Incubation period. The average incubation period varies from twenty-six to forty-two days.

Sequelae. The mortality rates are 1%–2% higher than in hepatitis A. In pregnant women, mortality rate is 10%–20%.

Transmission. HEV is transmitted via the fecal-oral route, predominantly through contaminated water and ingestion of raw shellfish. This virus is responsible for sporadic infections as well as large epidemics of acute viral hepatitis in developing countries. HEV infection in industrialized countries, including the United States, is more common than previously recognized. A study conducted in a large civilian, noninstitutionalized US population found an average anti-HEV IgG seroprevalence rate of 21%, with a strongly positive age-wise correlation. Unfortunately, to date, there are no methods developed in analyzing water and food for hepatitis E. There is no evidence for sexual transmission or for transmission by transfusion. Unlike the other hepatitis viruses, HEV has animal reservoirs; thus, nonhuman primates, cows, pigs, sheep, goats, deer, wild boars, cats, dogs, and rodents are susceptible to the HEV infection. In the United States and Sweden, studies on HEV prevalence among swine handlers and veterinarian workers have shown higher prevalence in these populations.

Treatment. There is no effective treatment hepatitis E. A balanced diet and bed rest are recommended.

Epidemiology. Hepatitis E is widespread in Southeast Asia, Northern and East Africa, India, and Central America. In 2004, there was an outbreak in Chad; with 1,442 cases reported, 46 people died. In Sudan, on the same year, there were 6,861 cases reported, and 87 people died. The disease is thought to be zoonosis. The high-risk population is military personnel of developing countries. There have been no reported cases of hepatitis E in the USA, although 2% of people tested had positive serological results. This makes many investigators question the validity of hepatitis E serological testing.

Prevention. Currently, there is no vaccine for hepatitis E. Improving sanitation is the most important measure.

Cultures. There is no reliable culture system for HEV, and nonhuman primates are the smallest animal models.

Historical reference. Hepatitis E had not been recognized until 1980; nevertheless, it was first documented in New Delhi in 1955 when twenty-nine thousand cases of icteric hepatitis occurred following contamination of drinking water. Initially, it had been thought that this outbreak had been due to an HAV infection, but retrospective analyzes of serum saved from that outbreak revealed HEV.

Family Togaviridae

Togaviridae encompasses Eastern equine encephalitis virus (EEEV), Western equine encephalitis virus (WEEV), and Venezuelan equine encephalitis virus (VEEV), viruses that belong to the genus *Alphaviruses*. The current classification of the genus *Alphavirus* includes twenty-nine different species with multiple subtypes and varieties represented within some species. Most viruses from the New World are neurotropic—they cause encephalitis in humans and in a variety of domesticated animals—while Old World alphaviruses ordinarily cause only an arthralgia and rash syndrome that is rarely life threatening. In the New World, the presence of the virus in mosquito salivary glands mediates the infection of vertebrates that serve as amplifying hosts, producing high-titer viremia until the virus is cleared by their immune system.

EEEV appears to be an anomaly among the alphaviruses in that this virus does not replicate well in lymphoid tissues but, nevertheless, achieves neuroinvasion and is highly neurovirulent. All alphaviruses are spherical and have a diameter of 60–65 nm. Superficial to the phospholipid bilayer, there is the outer layer consisting of a glycoprotein shell with protruding glycoprotein spikes. The nucleocapsid core contains the single-stranded RNA genome of over eleven thousand nucleotides in length. Alphaviruses replicate in the cytoplasm of infected cells after entry via receptor-mediated endocytosis.

Under unique ecological conditions, EEEV and WEEV are transmitted from avian hosts to dead-end hosts—equines and humans.

Eastern Equine Encephalitis

Eastern equine encephalitis (EEE) is a disease of wild birds that is transmitted to horses and humans (dead-end hosts) by mosquitoes. Sometimes the EEE virus is capable of crossing the blood-brain barrier, causing severe and often fatal acute encephalitis, an inflammation of the brain parenchyma.

Table 4.10

Properties of Eastern Equine Encephalitis Virus

Virion: spherical, 65–70 nm in diameter

Envelope: from cytoplasmic membrane

Capsid: icosahedral

Genome: +ssRNA, 11.7 kb

Target cell type: neurons

Reservoir: wading birds, pheasants, passerine songbirds, and starlings

Vector: 27 species of mosquitoes, predominantly *Aedes sollicitans*, *Aedes vexans*, *Coquillettidia*, *Culiseta melanura*, and *Culex* spp.

Diseases: Eastern equine encephalitis

Vaccine: none for humans

Signs and symptoms. EEE is characterized by a diffuse CNS involvement. EEEV has an infection rate of 33%. The type of illness depends on the age of the person as well as other host factors. Some people who become infected with EEEV may be asymptomatic. Systemic infection has an abrupt onset and is characterized by nonspecific signs and symptoms such as chills, fever, malaise, arthralgia, and myalgias. The prodromal phase is often short, averaging five to ten days, after which come headaches, irritability, restlessness, drowsiness, and vomiting, abdominal pains with diarrhea, cyanosis, convulsions, and coma. Death usually occurs two to ten days after onset of symptoms but can occur much later.

Diagnosis. Preliminary diagnosis is ordinarily based on the patient's clinical features, places and dates of travel, activities, and an epidemiologic history of the location where the infection occurred. Confirmation of clinical findings is usually accomplished by testing of serum or CSF to detect virus-specific IgM and neutralizing antibodies. In fatal cases, nucleic acid amplification, histopathology with immunohistochemistry, and virus culture of autopsy tissues are useful.

Incubation period. The incubation period for EEE ranges from four to ten days.

Sequelae. The prognosis in infected patients is extremely poor; 50%–70% of infected individuals die. Only 10% of patients fully recover. Surviving patients, especially children, are often profoundly affected by neurological and physical sequelae that include mental retardation, hemiparesis, aphasia, emotional instability, convulsions, hemiplegia, strabismus, impaired vision, partial deafness, and speech disorders.

Transmission. The alphavirus that causes EEE is found ordinarily in the mosquito subtype *C. melanura*, which breeds in freshwater swamps and feeds on passerine birds. Nevertheless, the EEE virus was isolated from twenty-seven other species of mosquitoes in the United States. The infected birds subsequently exhibit a high level of viremia, which differs from human and equine cases in which viremia is often low.

Treatment. There is no effective antiviral drug therapy.

Epidemiology. EEE occurs in Eastern and Southern United States, and its antigenic variant affects Mexico, South America, and the Caribbean. In the United States, Georgia, Louisiana, Massachusetts, New Jersey, and Florida have recorded the largest numbers of Eastern equine encephalitis cases. The virus found in North America is more pathogenic than the variant. EEE was first recognized in 1938. From 1955 to 1997, 256 cases, both sporadic and epidemic types, were reported to the US CDC. Approximately, 12–17 cases occur in the United States annually. There were only 4 in 1997. In 2003, an epidemic occurred in North Carolina where twenty-six cases were reported. The total confirmed number of cases as CDC reported in the United States is 220 between the years 1964 to 2004.

Most infections occur in summer or early fall; cases of EEE are almost nonexistent in winter months. An additional risk increase occurs during epizootic outbreaks among horses or caged birds.

Prevention. Vaccines to prevent EEE are available for horses, but none has been licensed for human use. Personal protection from mosquito bites is the only effective prevention strategy.

Cultures. In experimentally infected laboratory mice, EEEV produces a neurologic disease that resembles human and equine infections. The virus is detected in the brain as early as a day-one postinfection. Clinical signs of murine disease include ruffled hair, anorexia, vomiting, lethargy, posterior limb paralysis, convulsions, and coma.

Western Equine Encephalitis

The Western equine encephalitis (WEE) virus can cause disease in humans, horses, and some species of birds. WEE is an acute inflammation of the brain parenchyma, often with secondary meningeal involvement. The WEE virus is a member of the family Togaviridae, genus *Alphavirus*. The disease it causes is usually subclinical. It may mimic many viral and inflammatory syndromes such as flu-like illness or encephalitis. The prodromal phase is often short, averaging one to four days, and consists of fever, headache, chills, nausea, and vomiting.

Table 4.11
Properties of Western Equine Encephalitis Virus

Size: 70 nm in *diameter*
Virion: spherical
Envelope: from cytoplasmic membrane
Capsid: icosahedral

Genome: +ssRNA, 10–13 kb

Target cell type: neurons

Reservoir: domestic and passerine birds

Vector: mosquitoes *Culex tarsalis*

Transmission: mosquito bite

Diseases: Western equine encephalitis

Vaccine: none

Many adults may never develop any signs and symptoms besides the prodromal ones. Once neurologic symptoms arise, patients have a poorer prognosis and decompensate rapidly. Those symptoms include the following:

- Headache
- Confusion
- Sensory or motor loss
- Somnolence, a state of near-sleep, a strong desire for sleep
- Seizures
- Neck stiffness
- Photophobia

Focal necrosis is often found in the following areas:

- Striatum
- Globus pallidus
- Cerebral cortex
- Thalamus
- Pons
- Meninges

Neutrophils and macrophages may infiltrate the brain parenchyma and may cause neuronal destruction, neuronophagia, focal necrosis, and spotty demyelination. Cell death by apoptosis occurs primarily in the glial and inflammatory cells.

Diagnosis. WEE is difficult to diagnose because of the lack of specificity in symptoms. Differential diagnosis consists of a long list of neurodebilitating diseases, some of which include bartonellosis, cytomegalovirus virus infection, HSV infection, histoplasmosis, Lyme disease, mumps, EBV infection, and many others.

Incubation period. The initial symptoms may progress rapidly to CNS symptoms of mental confusion, somnolence, coma, and death in one to two days, or they may resolve without sequelae.

Sequelae. The primary complications, other than death, in WEE are the variable levels of CNS impairment. Patients with mild neurologic symptoms often rapidly recover, ordinarily with very few residual effects. Children who develop neurologic symptoms have a poorer prognosis. The fatality rate is 3%–4%.

Transmission. The virus cannot be transmitted via the aerosol route. It is spread by the mosquito *Culex tarsalis*, a primary vector of the disease. The mosquito prefers warm, moist environments and is often found on the West Coast of the United States and Canada. *C. tarsalis* are in close interactions with the native birds, which are reservoirs of the infection. This makes the infection endemic. No cases of bird transmission of the disease have been reported. Epidemic outbreaks in the equine or pheasant population often precede human epidemics of WEE. The virus can also be transferred transplacentally, causing massive cerebral necrosis and fetus death. Infection via contaminated blood transfusions is unlikely.

Treatment. There are no effective therapeutic drugs. Supportive care is the standard treatment. It includes intravenous fluids and medication to control fever and pain.

Epidemiology. The total confirmed number of cases of WEE in the United States, as CDC reported, is 639 between the years 1964 and 2004. WEE occurs primarily in Western United States and Canada. It is most common between April and September, with peaks in July and August, which is likely due to the peak of vector population during these periods. Adults are often targets of the vector. The infectivity rate is 1:1000. However, older adults tend to develop a more severe disease. The infectivity rate in infants is 1:1, so infection in infants is more common. It is also more common in males than in females, perhaps because of occupational exposure of rural land workers.

Prevention. There is no licensed vaccine for human use.

Cultures. The tissue cultures, usually used to observe viral growth, are green monkey kidneys, duck embryo fibroblasts, and *Aedes albopictus.*

Venezuelan Equine Encephalitis

Table 4.12
Properties of Venezuelan Equine Encephalitis virus

Size: 65–70 nm in diameter
Virion: spherical
Envelope: from cytoplasmic membrane
Capsid: icosahedral
Genome: +ssRNA, 11.5 kb
Target cell type: neurons
Vector: mosquitoes
Reservoir: vertebrates
Diseases: Venezuelan equine encephalitis

Venezuelan equine encephalitis (VEE) circulates in South America and Panama and has an ability to cause fatal disease in humans and horses. The disease manifests with the sudden onset of fever, chills, myalgia, prostration, arthralgia, retro-ocular pain, a headache of increasing severity, and decreased consciousness for several days. This is caused by exposure to mosquitoes infected with the Venezuelan equine encephalitis virus (VEEV) of the genus *Alphavirus*. Flu-like symptoms range from mild to severe, with prominent lymphoid and reticuloendothelial involvement. Development into neurological disease occurs in only 4%–14% of symptomatic cases. Fatalities are rare.

The person-to-person transmission is possible since VEEV has been isolated from the human pharynx and aerosol transmission of the virus has occurred as a result of laboratory accidents or lack of laboratory precautions. Until 1969, VEEV was one of seven standardized biological weapons developed in the United States. The virus remains a potentially potent biological weapon since it is relatively stable in the environment and can incapacitate thousands of people for a week or more and cause psychological stress to millions. Other than supportive care, no specific treatment is available for VEE. A live attenuated virus is used to vaccinate equines. A formalin-inactivated virus has been used to vaccinate human laboratory workers at risk, a vaccine not available to the general public.

West Nile Fever

The virus has had an important impact on human health in the United States because it took advantage of species that do well around people.

Marm Kilpatrick, University of California,
New York Times, July 15, 2012

West Nile fever (WNF) is an acute febrile disease with lymphadenopathy and maculopapular rash that used to be known to occur in Africa before it had been introduced to the United States. The causative agent is the West Nile virus (WNV), which is introduced to humans and other animals through an insect bite, producing viremia and a generalized systemic infection.

Table 4.13
Properties of West Nile Virus

Virion: spherical

Envelope: from cytoplasmic membrane

Capsid: icosahedral

Genome: +ssRNA

Target cell type: neurons

Reservoir: various birds, especially robins in the USA

Vector: insects, especially *Culex* mosquitoes

Susceptible hosts: humans; birds, especially crows; horses

Diseases: West Nile fever; one in 150 becomes severely ill with encephalitis

First human case West Nile district of Uganda, 1937; first USA case was in Queens in 1999

Vaccine: none

Signs and symptoms. A total of 80% of people infected with WNV are asymptomatic—in others, it may produce illness with severe symptoms such as high fever; headache; nausea; vomiting; swollen lymph glands; a skin rash on the chest, stomach, and back; neck stiffness; stupor; coma; tremors; convulsions; muscle weakness; vision loss; numbness; and paralysis. The symptoms may last for several weeks, and neurological effects may be permanent. Some people may develop a brief, WNF-like illness (early symptoms) before they develop a more severe disease. Patients may still be infected with the virus several years after recovering from their initial illness. It can remain in the kidneys for years, potentially leading to kidney failure.

Diagnosis. Clinical diagnosis is followed by a positive laboratory test for antibodies and antigens of WNV in the blood or CSF. Real-time

PCR is a molecular test that can quickly reveal the presence of the virus itself.

Incubation period. The incubation period ordinarily ranges from two to fifteen days.

Sequelae. Although not common, transitory meningeal involvement may occur during the acute stage. The virus may produce fatal encephalitis in older people who have a delayed antibody response.

Transmission. The WNV is introduced through the bite of a *Culex* mosquito that has picked up the virus by feeding on an infected bird. It produces viremia and a generalized systemic infection.

Treatment. There is no specific treatment for WNV infection except supportive care: possible hospitalization, administration of intravenous fluids, and respiratory support.

Epidemiology. West Nile virus was first detected in the United States in 1999 when it caused seven deaths. Since then, approximately twenty-five thousand human cases have been reported, causing more than one thousand deaths. It is normally spread as a mild infection in birds, but in 2003, a dead bird that was found in Kingwood, Texas, tested positive for West Nile virus, although American birds were not assumed to have fatal meningitis. As it turned out, the *Culex* mosquitoes were spreading the West Nile virus from infected birds to other animals, including humans, causing flu-like symptoms and, in some cases, encephalitis and meningitis that cause paralysis. The virus spread in the USA because its favored hosts are the American robin, whose ecological niches are lawns and agricultural fields. The American robin is known as a super spreader of the West Nile virus, though to be more accurate, it is the main reservoirs of the disease; the spreader, a vector, is a *Culex* mosquito, which finds robins especially appealing. Replication of the WNV in American robins begins when adult mosquitoes emerge in early spring and continues until fall. The West Nile season usually begins in mid-July and can continue through fall, depending on the weather; more human cases occur in July, August, and September than in other months. Humans and horses serve as incidental, dead-end hosts. The West Nile virus may be transmitted to mosquitoes by apparently healthy humans or animals. This possibility has the potential to start epidemics in new regions of the world.

Prevention. Mosquito abatement is a logical control measure. Residents in mosquito-prone areas are advised to wear protective clothing, such as long-sleeved shirts and pants from dusk until dawn, and to use a mosquito repellent, and to avoid wearing perfume or cologne which can attract mosquitoes.

Cultures. In the laboratory conditions, the virus propagates in chick embryo and tissue cultures, producing plaques on cell monolayers.

German Measles (Rubella)

Table 4.14
Properties of Rubella Virus

Virion: spherical
Envelope: loose lipid envelope from cytoplasmic membrane
Capsid: icosahedral
Genome: +ssRNA, 10 kb
Reservoir: humans only
Transmission: person-to-person contact, aerosols
Vector: no insect vector
Target cell type: vascular endothelial cells
Transmission: droplet contact
Diseases: German measles (rubella)

Symptoms: mild disease with a macular rash resembling measles but less extensive; it disappears in three days
Diagnosis: acute IgM, acute/convalescent IgG
Therapy: no antivirals; supportive care
Vaccine: attenuated virus (mumps, measles, and rubella [MMR])

German measles or rubella is an acute viral disease that causes fever and rash in children and is also known as three-day measles. It is caused by the rubella virus.

Signs and symptoms. Rubella infection of children and adults is usually mild, self limiting, and often asymptomatic.

Diagnosis. The rubella virus–specific antibodies are present in people recently infected by the German measles. The diagnosis is confirmed with a clinical manifestation of the characteristic rash.

Incubation period. Ordinarily, incubation time is of two to three weeks.

Sequelae. There is about a 35% incidence of serious fetal damage in pregnant women infected with German measles. The malformations include the following:

- Heart defects
- Eye cataracts
- Deaf-mutism, a state of being both unable to hear and unable to speak
- Mental retardation
- Death

In neonates with congenital rubella, there may be a single serious defect or multiple ones; 15% die during their first year.

Transmission. Transmission is airborne, from person to person. The disease is often spread from asymptomatic carriers. From the mother's blood, the rubella virus crosses the placenta into developing tissues of the fetus. It can persist throughout gestation and into the neonatal period. The fetus is infected at the same time as the mother, resulting in malformations.

Treatment. There is no specific treatment for rubella except supportive care. Treatment of congenital rubella in neonates is focused on management of the complications.

Epidemiology. Since the vaccine was introduced, there has been a drastic reduction in the number of cases of rubella in the USA and other developed countries.

Not to be confused with
German measles = Rubella =
= Togaviridae = +ssRNA
Measles = Rubeola =
= Paramyxoviridae = - ssRNA

Figure 4.5. German measles vs. measles

Prevention. The attenuated virus is routinely given to children as part of a mumps, measles, and rubella vaccination (MMR). WHO recommends the first dose is given at twelve to eighteen months of age, with a second dose at thirty-six months. The vaccination is recommended for women of childbearing age as well as certain health-care personnel who are seronegative.

Cultures. The virus is isolated from throat washing and the blood of patients. It more readily grows in green monkey kidney cells in which it multiplies without causing cytopathic effects. Rubella virus prevents destruction of the culture by the challenge of another virus such as picornaviruses or with arboviruses. The virus also grows in cells agglutinates of a day-old chick or adult goose erythrocytes. It is viable after storage for long periods, at least two years, at -70°C.

Family Coronaviridae

Coronaviridae are a group of enveloped, positive-strand RNA viruses of the group Nidovirales. Five different strains of Coronaviridae infect humans mainly in the winter and early spring seasons:

- HCoV-229E
- HCoV-OC43
- SARS-CoV (2002)
- NL63, NL, or the New Haven coronavirus (2004)
- HKU1 (2005)

They cause a significant portion of all common colds in human adults, primarily having an affinity to the upper respiratory and gastrointestinal tract.

Table 4.15
Properties of Coronaviridae

Size: 100–140 nm in diameter; 20 nm club-shaped surface spikes

Virion: pleomorphic

Envelope: from endoplasmic reticulum and Golgi membranes

Capsid: helical

Genome: +ssRNA, 26–33 kb

Target cell type: respiratory epithelium

Transmission: droplets from the respiratory secretions
Diseases: common cold, rhinitis, SARS
Discovered: 1960s

Coronaviruses are generally highly species-specific. In immunocompetent hosts, infection elicits neutralizing antibodies and cell-mediated immune responses that kill infected cells. It seems that Coronaviridae have recently emerged through zoonotic transmission to become a serious human pathogen.

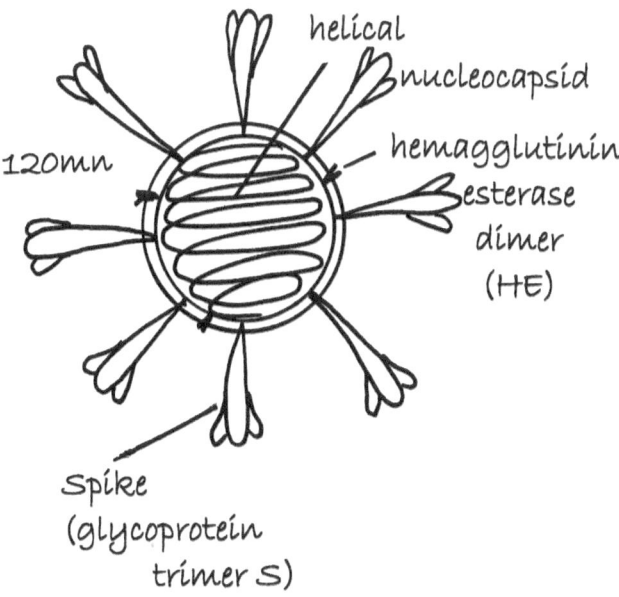

Figure 4.6. Architecture of Coronaviridae (corona = "crown" L). HE protein appears to play a role in binding to or release from the target cell. However, the precise function of HE protein and of its enzymatic activity remains poorly understood.

Severe Acute Respiratory Syndrome

Table 4.16
Properties of SARS

Size: 60 –130 nm
Virion: pleomorphic
Envelope: M protein is the major component
Capsid: helical
Genome: +ssRNA
Target cell type: respiratory epithelium
Transmission: droplets from the respiratory secretions; less frequent: fecal or airborne transmission
Reservoir: horseshoe bats, palm civets (*Paguma larvata*)
Diseases: Severe acute respiratory syndrome (SARS)
First human case: Guangdong Province, China, 2003
Vaccine: none

Severe acute respiratory syndrome (SARS) is an influenza-like illness with fever, dry cough, myalgias, and in some patients with diarrhea. The pathogenic agent responsible for SARS in humans and civets is the SARS coronavirus (SARS-CoV). The unique feature of SARS-CoV is that it, unlike the other members of the family, causes both upper and lower respiratory tract infections and can also cause gastroenteritis. Indeed, despite the similarity with a genome organization to other Coronaviridae, the SARS-CoV RNA sequence is only distantly related to that group. Whether the SARS-CoV has "jumped" from a nonhuman host reservoir to humans, the molecular basis of such a jump remains an unanswered question.

Signs and symptoms. Breath sounds upon auscultation resembles that produced with viral influenza, and X- rays show characteristic of viral pneumonia; it is quiet without rales. Other signs and symptoms are similar to influenza:

- Fever (38°C)
- Myalgias
- Dyspnea, a shortness of breath

It is a biphasic infection, meaning the fever decreases after few days and the patient improves, then fever recurs in another few days. Leucocyte and platelet counts are usually normal or slightly decreased. It is often confused with the viral influenza A, Legionnaires' disease, and tularemic pneumonia. Laboratory diagnosis is achieved by viral isolation or specific SARS serology.

Incubation period. SARS is characterized by a long incubation period—six days.

Transmission. SARS, in contrast to diseases like flu or rubella, is only moderately transmissible. It is predominantly spread in droplets that are shed from the respiratory secretions of infected persons. Fecal or airborne transmission seems to be less frequent. There is no direct evidence of transmission from an asymptomatic person.

Epidemiology. The first case was registered in 2003 in the province of Guangdong, China. Because of global travel, it spread quickly from China to twenty-five countries, causing more than seven hundred deaths. Many of its victims were medical personnel. On three occasions, SARS virus escaped from laboratories where it was being studied. The outbreak was contained, and since 2004, no new cases have been reported.

Treatment. There is no effective medication against SARS virus. Routine treatment includes a prescription of antibiotics such as quinolones and macrolides because of their immunomodulatory properties. Immunomodulator is a substance that adjusts the immune response to a desired level by augmenting the ability of the immune system to produce antibodies or sensitized cells that recognize and react with the antigen that initiated their production. During the

SARS outbreak, there were various antiviral medications prescribed despite the lack of evidence about their effectiveness.

Cultures. Some biologic features of the SARS-CoV *in vitro* differ from those of other coronaviruses. SARS-CoV has a peculiar tropism for Vero cells, a continuous cell line established from monkey kidney epithelial cells. It is capable of growing at 37°C while other members of Coronaviridae grow at lower temperatures. Another striking peculiarity that has been mentioned earlier is its ability to infect lower respiratory tract tissues.

Historical reference. In February 12, 2003, China first reported 305 cases of an atypical pneumonia to WHO, which immediately issued emergency travel alert and named the illness SARS. Scientists all over the world agreed to unprecedented cooperation. Credit for the coronavirus findings, which definitively pinpoints the cause of SARS, is attributed to the thirteen laboratories, working in conjunction with WHO. In April 12, 2003, Canadian scientists in Vancouver posted the complete genome of SARS on the Internet.

Family Retroviridae

Table 4.17
Properties of family Retroviridae

Size: 80–130 nm in diameter
Virion: spherical, carry the reverse transcriptase and integrase proteins
Envelope: from cytoplasmic membrane
Capsid: helical
Genome: ssRNA, 7–10 kb
Target cell type: macrophages, CD4+ and CD8+ T lymphocytes,
B lymphocytes

Transmission: neonatal infection, sexual transmission, blood

Diseases: AIDS, simian AIDS, FAIDS

Discovered by Vilhelm Ellermann and Oluf Bang in 1908

The members of this large group of viruses use a retrograde flow of information from RNA to DNA instead of from DNA to RNA and, thus, break the rule of the central dogma. Hundreds of those viruses had been studied in higher vertebrates though there are those that infect fish and invertebrates as well. The electron microscopy observations reveal that the different genera of the family Retroviridae differ in their structure, but all retroviruses encode four genes in the following order:

- *Gag*, a gene that provides the basic physical infrastructure of the virus
- *Pro*, a gene that encodes a protease that is required for the processing of *gag*
- *Pol*, a gene that encodes for three activities: (1) reverse transcriptase, (2) RNase H, and (3) integrase
- *Env*, a gene that encodes the envelope glycoproteins present at the surface of the enveloped retrovirion

The genome of the Retroviridae is diploid, which consists of two copies of ssRNA that are normally identical. Why it is so is not clear since, as was shown in *in vitro* studies, retroviral reverse transcriptase can use only a single copy of the RNA to produce a dsDNA. Perhaps during infection *in vivo*, the process is more efficient. It is also possible that there are advantages of the diploidy—for example, overcoming the same damages in the RNA by switching templates, opening opportunities to recombination that, as we know, occurs frequently in retroviruses. Another characteristics of retroviruses is that their ssRNA is capped and polyadenylated, meaning having a tail that has only adenine bases. This tail is called a polyadenylic acid tail.

HIV:

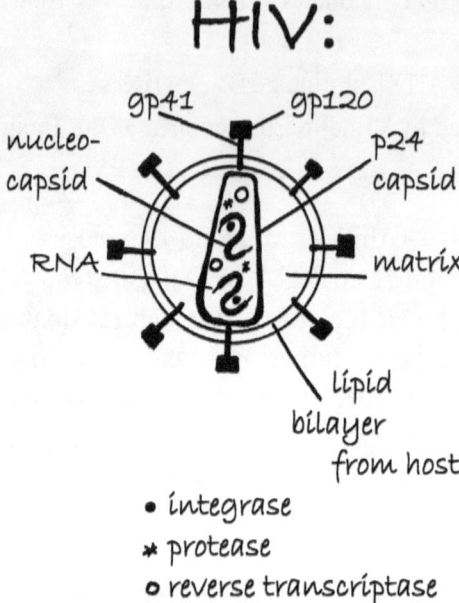

Figure 4.7. Architecture of HIV

Retroviruses are differentiated into simple and complex viruses, depending on their genomes. Simple viruses are viruses that have only the genes mentioned above while complex viruses contain a number of regulatory genes (three to six genes) in addition to those four basic genes. The regulatory genes allow complex viruses to regulate the development of the infection cycle. Specific functions include the following:

- Transport across the nuclear membrane of subviral particles
- Activation of the transcription of the provirus
- Export of viral RNA to the cytoplasm
- Promotion of virus assembly

All the above support more vigorous viral replication, which can be fatal to the host cell. Three known genera—*Deltaretrovirus*, *Lentivirus*, and S*pumavirus*—are complex viruses while the rest are simple retroviruses. Members of *Deltaretrovirus* and *Lentivirus* genera encompass human pathogens:

- Deltaretroviruses cause B cell lymphoma, T cell lymphoma, and neurological disorders; the transmission occurs through mother's milk, sexual intercourse, and blood transmission.
- Lentiviruses, HIV-1 and HIV-2, cause AIDS; the routes of transmission is the same as with deltaretroviruses.

HIV-1 is capable of replicating to a high titer in some cell types, with the result that cells become destroyed. The simple viruses do not kill the host cell but establish a persistent infection. Lentiviruses establish a lifelong, chronic infection that elicits a strong immune response that is still unable to clear the infection (table 4.18).

Table 4.18
Viruses of Genus *Lentiviruses*

Virus and Disease	Abbreviation	Hosts
*Human immunodeficiency virus 1*AIDS	HIV-1	Humans
Human immunodeficiency virus 2 AIDS	HIV-2	Humans
Simian immunodeficiency virus Simian AIDS	SIV	Monkeys
Feline immunodeficiency virus FAIDS	FIV	Cats
Bovine immunodeficiency virus Jembrana	BIV	Cattle
Visna virus Neurological	–	Sheep
Equine infectious anemia virus Anemia	EIAV	Horses
Caprine arthritis encephalitis virus	CAEV	Goats

Acquired Immunodeficiency Syndrome

Ending the AIDS epidemic is likely to be far more complicated than ending most other epidemics.

—Altman, L. K., *New York Times*, July 31, 2012

Table 4.19
Properties of HIV-1 and HIV-2

Size: 80–100 nm in diameter

Virion: spherical, carry the reverse transcriptase and integrase proteins

Envelope: from cytoplasmic membrane

Capsid: helical

Genome: ssRNA, 7–10 kb

Target cell type: macrophages, CD4+ T lymphocytes, microglial cells

Transmission: neonatal infection, sexual transmission, blood

Diseases: Human immunodeficiency virus (HIV) infection and AIDS

Discovered in 1983 by Luc Montagnier and his colleagues at the Pasteur

Institute

The two human lentiviruses, HIV-1 and HIV-2, cause the well-known disease called acquired immunodeficiency syndrome (AIDS). The HIV-2 is not as serious an infection as HIV-1 since its latent period is much longer and the virus is not as easily transmissible as HIV-1. Both viruses target macrophages and CD4+ T cells, also called T4 cells, in humans. CD4 is a primary receptor for all human lentiviruses. This receptor alone is not enough to establish the HIV infection.

Chemokine coreceptors, either CCR5 or CXCR4, are required for the entry of the virus, as was discussed earlier, into the target cell. HIV-1 is divided into three distinct groups—M, N, O—and subtype/clade—A to K. While the most studied group is HIV-1B, it is the HIV-1C group that has caused millions of deaths among half the infected people in the world. HIV-1C differs from HIV-1B by the rates of genomic variation and different patterns of drug-resistant mutations. People with HIV-1C infection may be "hypertransmitters," who are more highly infectious to their sexual contacts. Antiretroviral drug treatment (ART) dramatically decreases the viral load and HIV transmission.

Signs and symptoms. Primary infection may be asymptomatic or accompanied by nonspecific symptoms that usually appear three to six weeks after an infection. Symptoms may include the following:

- Rash
- Fever
- Diarrhea
- Arthralgias
- Myalgias
- Nausea
- Sore throat
- Cough and shortness of breath
- Lethargy
- Headache
- Stiff neck
- Night sweats

During this phase, the number of CD4+ T cells declines and an immune response is mounted when antibodies are produced and the number of both the CD8+ cytotoxic T cells (CTLs) is increased. Such an immune response reduces the amount of virus in the blood while the number of CD4+ recovers but does not reach a preinfection level. The symptoms of disease at this point improve, and the infection becomes latent as the virus continues to replicate actively, particularly in lymph nodes. The immune system continues to fight the infection, which produces 10^8–10^9 virus particles per day, releasing them into the peripheral blood supply. In untreated individuals, it eventually leads to a steady decline in the number of CD4+ T cells. With time, the immune system becomes overwhelmed with the escalating number of viruses and becomes incapable of dealing with the wide range of opportunistic infections. This happens when the number of CD4+ T cells drops below 500 cells/µl. This manifests with clinical signs and symptoms such as generalized lymphadenopathy, headache, fever, malaise, and weight loss. The reactivation of the herpes zoster virus and the molluscum contagiosum virus is manifested as skin lesions outbreak. One of the most characteristic signs is the appearance of an oral thrush, creamy white lesions usually on the tongue or inner cheeks. This is caused by the overgrown fungus *Candida albicans*. Reactivation of *Mycobacterium tuberculosis* with an onset of tuberculosis is another side effect of the declination of CD4+ T cells.

One is diagnosed with AIDS when the numbers of CD4+ T cells drop lower than 200 cells/µl and to the signs and symptoms listed above and when diarrhea, caused by the invasion and growth of such protozoans as *Isospora belli* and *Cryptosporidia*, disseminated toxoplasma, become apparent. The bacterial infections with *Salmonella*, *Streptococci*, and *Haemophilus* are common. CNS infection with fungus *Cryptococcus neoformans* is a common cause of death in people with AIDS as well as the pneumonia caused by the yeast-like fungus *Pneumocystis*. Moreover, the characteristic cancers, such as B cell lymphoma (Epstein-Barr virus), Kaposi's sarcoma (HHV-8), and anogenital carcinoma (HPV), become apparent as well. Genital herpesviruses and cytomegaloviruses cause disseminated diseases of the lungs, the brains, etc. A wasting syndrome—diarrhea and malabsorption—is characteristic of a late-stage HIV infection. Whether it is caused by the HIV infection itself or opportunistic infections of the gut is unclear. Two-thirds of infected individuals develop an encephalopathy induced by the HIV infection itself, which is called AIDS dementia complex. The symptoms include dementia, motor and behavioral abnormalities, and seizures. In the brain tissue, HIV is present in macrophages and microglia but does not infect neurons.

The time of progression to AIDS following the infection by HIV is variable, depending on the strain of HIV and strength of the immune response against the virus, but averages about ten years. Once the symptoms of AIDS appear, the time to death is ordinarily one to two years, unless antiviral treatment is administrated.

Transmission. HIV is spread sexually, through contaminated blood (horizontal transmission), and from mother to child (vertical transmission).

Sexual transmission. The majority of HIV-1 infections result from seminal transmission, though the virus is also present in vaginal secretions of infected women. The probability of women becoming infected during unprotected vaginal intercourse with an infected male is 1/50 while the risk of a man becoming infected during heterosexual intercourse is less. Of course, the risk is much higher if genital lesions resulting from STDs are present. Also, the risk of infection is high during receptive anal intercourse. The virus can enter the host through mouth sores or small tears that sometimes develop in the rectum or vagina during sexual activity. The use of condoms reduces the risk of HIV transmission. An HIV-infected individual is 96% less likely to transmit the virus to their partners if they take antiretroviral drugs (ARVs).

Blood-borne transmission. The transmission by contaminated blood occurs via blood transfusions, the use of contaminated products by hemophiliacs, by a needlestick injury in health-care workers, and the sharing of needles by injecting drug users or via tattoo needles. The use of blood tests and screening of donors with risk factors have significantly reduced the transmission of HIV through blood products in developed countries.

Vertical transmission. One-fourth of the time, infected women transmit HIV to a newborn. Transmission occurs during delivery. The use of antiviral drugs has reduced transmission to infants in countries where the drugs are available. The breast milk of HIV-infected mothers contains reservoirs of HIV even when they are successfully treated with antiretroviral therapy.

Epidemiology. At the end of 1999, forty-three million people worldwide were living with HIV/AIDS; this total number has changed, and as of 2010, thirty-four million people are infected with HIV.

This incidence has changed little since 2004. It is estimated that 68% of all people in the world living with HIV are in the sub-Saharan

Africa—22.9 million, 1.9 million of whom are children. In some large cities in sub-Saharan Africa, 20%–40% of adults may be infected. The second highest regional HIV prevalence after sub-Saharan Africa is in the Caribbean, where adult prevalence of the disease is 0.9% compared to 5% in sub-Saharan Africa. More than half of all cases of HIV infection in North America and Western and Central Europe are in the USA—1.2 million. According to CDC estimation, 60% of HIV-positive youth in the USA have no idea they carry the HIV. New infections occur disproportionally among youth of color, who represent 80% of new infections. In most regions, the epidemics of HIV infection are stabilized. However, AIDS-related deaths continue to rise in Eastern Europe and Central Asia.

Table 4.20
Prevalence of the HIV Infection Around the World, 2010
(Data from UNAIDS World AIDS Day Report, 2011)

Worldwide: 34 million people are infected

Sub-Saharan Africa: 22.9 million people living with HIV

Caribbean: 200,000 people living with HIV, second highest regional HIV prevalence after sub-Saharan Africa

South and Southeast Asia: 4 million people living with HIV; 270,000 new HIV infections, 40% less than at the epidemic's peak in 1996

Eastern Europe and Central Asia: 1.5 million people living with HIV; 250% increase in the number of people living with HIV (2001–2010)

India: new HIV infections fell by 56%; still the largest number of people living with HIV in Asia

China: disproportional distribution; 53% of people with HIV live in five provinces

Indonesia: disproportional distribution; most people with HIV live in Papua and West Papua provinces

Middle East and North Africa: AIDS-related deaths are on the rise in some countries while in others, the epidemic is stable

Latin America: 1.5 million people living with HIV; the HIV epidemics are stable; considerable decrease in new HIV infections and AIDS-related deaths among children

Oceania: 54,000 people live with HIV

Russian Federation and Ukraine: account for almost 90% of the Eastern Europe and the Central Asia

North America and Western and Central Europe: 2.2 million people

USA: 1.2 million

Prevention and treatment. There's no cure for HIV/AIDS, but there are antiretroviral drug combination that can prevent HIV-infected women from passing the infection to their newborns. There is also medication to dramatically slow the progress of the disease and prevent infection among HIV adults. About 800,000 of the 1.2 million HIV-infected people in the USA alone are thought to fall somewhere along the continuum of disengagement. There is no vaccine that will prevent HIV infection. Currently, only public education to slow the spread of the disease and the development of antiviral drugs has had any success in controlling the virus. The safe-sex practices, such as the use of condoms, have lowered the number of new infections, especially among gay white males. Education campaigns in many developing countries have succeeded in slowing the spread of the disease. Still, they do not stop it and will never succeed in eliminating the virus from the population. Creating an AIDS-free generation even through a cure and a vaccine is still a distant hope.

CHAPTER V

Negative Single-Stranded RNA Viruses

Outline

Family Orthomyxoviridae

Orthomyxoviridae contain influenza viruses. Many of the members of the family are quite susceptible to antibody immunity and vaccination.

Viral Influenza (Flu)

Table 5.1
Properties of Influenza Viruses

Size: 80–120 nm

Virion: spherical

Envelope: from cytoplasmic membrane

Capsid: helical

Genome: -ssRNA, 8 segments, 10 genes

Sentinel host: human

Target cell type: ciliated cells of the respiratory mucosa

Transmission: airborne or droplet, direct or indirect

Reservoir: humans, birds, mammals

Treatment: supportive care

Diseases: viral influenza

Vaccine: attenuated (nasal spray), subunit/conjugate (injection)

Influenza is an acute, highly communicable respiratory tract infection that is characterized by an explosive onset, the rapid spread, and involvement of a high frequency of serious secondary bronchopneumonia. There are three major types of influenza viruses:

• Influenza virus A
• Influenza virus B
• Influenza virus C

Influenza A and B are the most important human pathogens, with A being the most severe. Over 90% of influenza is caused by the influenza A virus and 10% by the influenza B virus. The influenza virus C does not cause typical influenza but may cause a mild upper respiratory tract infection in children and adults. In addition to human types, the influenza A strains may also affect pigs, horses, ducks, and chicken.

Influenza viruses that affect humans first establish a local upper respiratory tract infection. They target and kill mucus-secreting epithelial cells. Later, the viruses are capable of spreading down to the lower respiratory tract, where they cause shedding of bronchial and alveolar epithelium down to the basement membrane. Gas exchange becomes compromised, and breathing becomes difficult. Because the primary line of defense is compromised, patients with influenza are very susceptible to superinfections, especially with *Haemophilus influenzae.*

A fascinating attribute of the influenza viruses is the ability to produce epidemics and pandemics. Antigenic changes appear to be continually taking place; the influenza virus has a mutation rate about one hundred times greater than many other viruses. This characteristic is mainly determined by its peculiar viral ultrastructure. First of all, the influenza virus is an RNA virus, and unlike the DNA viruses, it cannot correct copying errors during the process of replication. Second, the influenza virus has a segmented genome with each of eight loosely bound segments responsible for producing one or two viral proteins. The loose connection between segments allows them to come apart and rearrange with segments from other nearby viruses. If they combine with segments from viruses in other animals, there can be major changes to the surface antigens, a phenomenon known as an antigenic shift. This will make a new virus completely unrecognized by the human immune system it encounters. Another factor that increases the possibilities of various mutations is dense populations. Asia is a major site of an antigenic shift because of very high population densities.

Chickens, pigs, and ducks are excellent reservoirs for the virus as they harbor the virus but do not get sick from it. In China, they are commonly raised together; all are likely to get infected with human flu virus, and if they are concurrently harboring the virus from their own species, the viral reassortment may occur. With the recent increase in fish farming in China, which involves feeding hen feces to pigs and fertilizing the fishponds, which are also duck ponds with pig manure, there is cause for serious concern that the frequency of gene reassortment will increase over the next few years.

NA:

—disrupts the host's mucin barrier

HA:

—binds to the host's cell sialic acid

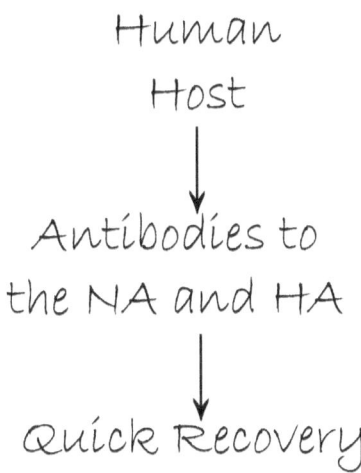

Human

Host

↓

Antibodies to
the NA and HA

↓

Quick Recovery

Figure 5.1. Neuraminidase (NA) and hemagglutinin (HA)

Orthomyxoviridae:
Influenza Nomenclature

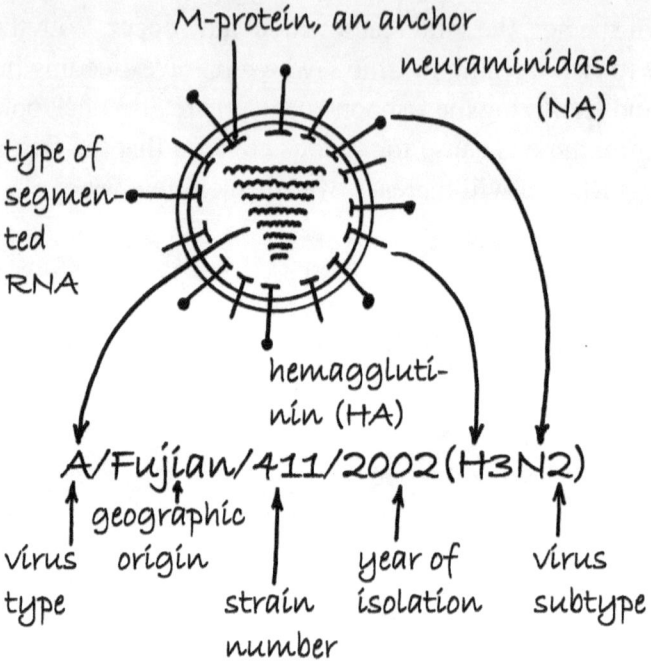

Figure 5.2. Influenza nomenclature

Signs and symptoms. Inflammation of the respiratory tract is the usual extent of pathology. The signs and symptoms include the following:

- Chills
- Malaise
- Fever
- Myalgias
- Profound prostration

Respiratory symptoms may occur but are not pathognomonic. Patients with primary influenza pneumonia usually present a dry cough that may be blood tinged. Severities of the pandemics are determined by the development of pneumonia often of bacterial etiology. Purulent sputum indicates superimposed bacterial pneumonia. Sporadic cases are almost impossible to diagnose solely on clinical grounds.

Diagnosis. Rapid influenza tests for diagnosis include PCR, ELISA type assays, or immunofluorescence. Cultures can be useful to identify which subtype of influenza is causing the infections, which is important for public health authorities to know.

Incubation period. The incubation period is only one to four days.

Sequelae. Pneumonia, when it occurs, may be followed by death. Autopsies on victims reveal interstitial inflammation with necrosis of bronchiolar and alveolar epithelium. Histological examinations demonstrate that the viruses cause necrosis of the ciliated and goblet cells of the tracheal and bronchial mucosa but does not affect the basal layer of the epithelium.

Transmission. The disease is spread by direct and indirect contact, including droplet infection. The virus enters the body by the mouth and nose in airborne droplets and leaves by the same route. The drier air of winter facilitates the spread of the virus as the moist particles expelled by sneezes and coughs become dry very quickly, helping the virus to remain airborne for longer time. Therefore, influenza epidemics peak during the winter months.

The explosive outbreaks of an epidemic occur because of the high communicability of the disease, the large number of susceptible people, and the fact that during the early days of the attack, the patient is not confined to bed but mingles freely with other people. The virus is present in the nasopharynx from one to two days before to one to two days after the onset of symptoms. Epidemic occurs upon the emergence of a new strain since the influenza virus has a dramatic tendency to change its chemical and genetic nature.

Treatment. Mild to moderate influenza A or B may be treated with neuraminidase inhibitors (oseltamivir, zanamivir), which reduce symptoms in two days.

Epidemiology. Influenza is the most common cause of viral pneumonia. Millions of people are typically infected by an influenza virus each year in the USA, causing twenty thousand to forty thousand deaths annually, and 10% of those who develop pneumonia due to influenza virus complication die. *Haemophilus influenzae,* staphylococci, pneumococci, and streptococci are important secondary invaders in this and other respiratory diseases.

Cultures. Among laboratory animals, ferrets are more susceptible than other species. Several passages in mice increase its virulence for this animal, producing extensive pulmonary consolidation and death. The developing chick embryo readily supports the growth of the virus, but for most strains, even a high level of infection fails to produce glossy detectable lesions. The virus-infected bacteria burst upon virus liberation. In tissue culture, the infected cells do not burst while liberating all the influenza viruses that they contain. A single infected cell produces about 60–120 virions, liberating them over a three-hour period in the first viral cycle. Histological examination does not reveal any damage to the cells at the first viral liberation.

Historical reference. The name *influenza* comes from Italian astrologers who centuries ago believed that the periodic appearance of the disease was in some way related to the "influence" of the heavenly bodies. An estimated twenty to forty million people worldwide died of the influenza in the pandemic of 1918. At that time, influenza was thought to be of bacterial etiology. Only in 1933 was it established that the etiological agent was a virus.

Family Paramyxoviridae

Table 5.2
Properties of Paramyxoviridae

Virion: spherical, 150–350 nm
Envelope: from cytoplasmic membrane
Capsid: helical
Genome: -ssRNA, 15–20 kb, 6–10 genes
Sentinel host: human
Reservoir: birds
Transmission: contact through conjunctiva
Diseases: mumps, measles, respiratory syncytial virus infection, parainfluenza, Nipah virus encephalitis, Hendra virus encephalitis

---

The Paramyxoviridae family is one of the largest and most rapidly growing groups of viruses causing significant human and veterinary diseases. The parainfluenza and respiratory syncytial viruses are responsible for the most cases of croup, bronchiolitis, and pneumonia in infants.

They are pleomorphic enveloped viruses in which the envelope is extremely fragile. They differ from the Orthomyxoviridae family in their slightly larger size and in their tendency to lyse as well as agglutinate erythrocytes. They also share few antigenic sites with the influenza virus. Unlike Orthomyxoviridae, Paramyxoviridae grows poorly in embryonated eggs. They grow well in primary monkey or human epithelial cell culture.

Mumps

Table 5.3
Properties of Mumps Virus

Virion: spherical, 150–350 nm

Envelope: from cytoplasmic membrane

Capsid: helical

Genome: -ssRNA, 15–20 kb, 7 genes

Transmission: direct contact

Reservoir: humans only

Diseases: mumps

Complications: pancreatitis, oophoritis, encephalitis, thyroiditis

Vaccine: attenuated virus

Mumps is a contagious viral infection, usually in children, that causes painful swelling of the parotid glands. *Epidemic parotitis* is another name for mumps. The etiologic agent is a single-stranded, negative-sense RNA virus from the family Paramyxoviridae and the genus *Rubulavirus*. Its genome is linear and consists of 15,384 nucleotides. The mumps virus enters via the respiratory tract, multiplies, invades the blood, and can affect many organs in addition to the salivary glands.

Signs and symptoms. Prodromal signs and symptoms of mumps are nonspecific and include low-grade fever, headache, muscle aches, stiff neck, malaise, and loss of appetite. Those signs and symptoms are followed by inflammation of salivary glands, an especially painful inflammation of the parotid gland (parotitis). It may occur on one (unilateral) or both (bilateral) sides. Other signs and symptoms may include dry mouth and swollen face and ears. Interestingly, 20% of people infected with mumps do not have classical signs and symptoms for mumps; instead, they develop upper respiratory infections similar to a common cold.

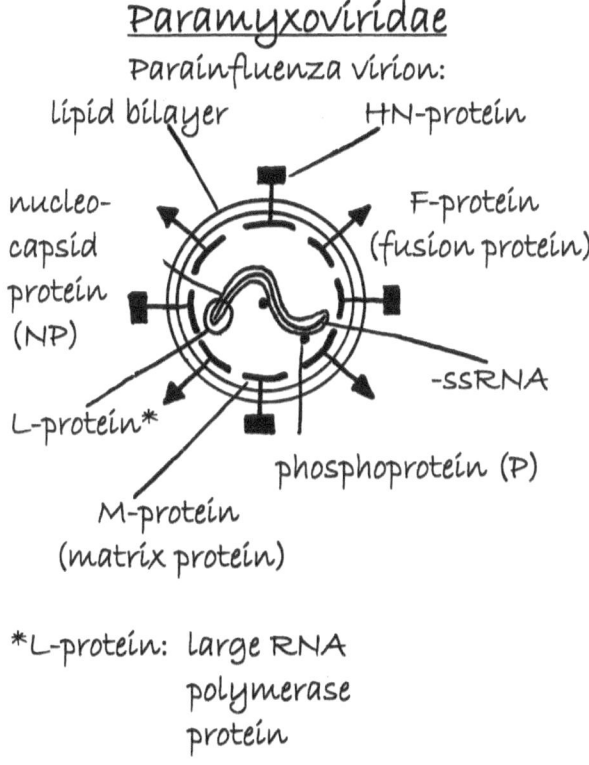

Paramyxoviridae
Parainfluenza virion:

lipid bilayer   HN-protein

nucleo-
capsid   F-protein
protein   (fusion protein)
(NP)

L-protein*   -ssRNA

phosphoprotein (P)

M-protein
(matrix protein)

*L-protein: large RNA
polymerase
protein

Figure 5.3. Architecture of parainfluenza virion

Incubation period. The time between infection and the clinical appearance of the signs and symptoms is between twelve to twenty-five days.

Sequelae. Severe complications are rare. Nevertheless, mumps may cause meningitis (10% risk), encephalitis (1.7%), orchitis (inflammation of the testes—30% risk), oophoritis (inflammation of the ovaries—5% risk), mastitis (inflammation of the breasts—31%), pancreatitis (4%), spontaneous abortion (in 27% of cases during the first trimester of pregnancy), and permanent deafness (0.005%).

Diagnoses. Clinical manifestations are sufficient for the diagnosis of mumps. The acute meningoencephalitis serology is the method of choice in confirming the infection. This method demonstrates the presence of specific IgM.

Transmission. Mumps is transmitted by direct contact with the saliva from an infected individual who coughs or sneezes.

Epidemiology. The number of cases decreased dramatically in the United States following the introduction of the mumps vaccine in 1967. From one hundred thousand to two hundred thousand cases to fewer than three hundred were reported in 2003. Recently, there has been increase in mumps in the USA. In 2006, there were six thousand cases reported across the nation. To date, there are fewer than one thousand cases annually. Infection is more common during late winter and spring. People with mumps are usually contagious one week before and two weeks after onset of the symptoms. Immunity acquired after contracting the disease is usually long-term. Reinfection is possible but is usually mild and atypical. The mumps virus affects only humans and is less contagious than measles and chicken pox. Infections are more common in schools, military headquarters, and orphanages.

Treatment. There is no specific treatment for mumps. Comfort care is required. The disease is self-limiting, running its course before receding.

Prevention. The most effective control measure is vaccination. Mumps vaccine is included in the MMR vaccine (measles, mumps, and rubella). The first dose is given at between twelve and fifteen months, and the second dose is given between four and six years of age. If one does not know if he or she was vaccinated, vaccination is still recommended.

Cultures. Monkey kidney cells in culture are more sensitive than embryonated eggs to human strains of mumps. Chick embryo tissues are used for growing mumps virus *in vitro*. The virus presented in inoculated tubes may be detected in two to five days by adsorption of chicken or guinea pig red cells by the infected cells.

Historical reference. Mumps was first described in the fifth century BC by Hippocrates. Although in modern times, mumps is considered to be a disease of childhood, historically, mumps was known as a disease affecting armies. Our understanding of mumps began in the eighteenth and nineteenth century. A high incident number among Soviet military recruits and in the US forces in Korea was reported. Serological surveys show that on average, 12%–16% of US military recruits entering training during 1989 and 1990 were susceptible to mumps.

The mumps virus was discovered in 1934 by two American scientists, Ernest William Goodpasture and Claude D. Johnson. Ten years later, German biologist Karl Habel and American biologist John Enders cultivated the virus in a chick embryo. Live attenuated mumps virus vaccines were developed in the 1960s in both the Soviet Union and the United States.

Measles (Rubeola)

Table 5.4
Properties of Rubeola Virus

Size: 100–200 nm
Virion: spherical
Envelope: from cytoplasmic membrane
Capsid: helical
Genome: -ssRNA
Target cell type: respiratory epithelium, lymphatic cells
Transmission: droplet contact
Diseases: measles, rash, coryza, and conjunctivitis

Complications: otitis media, pneumonia, encephalitis
Diagnosis: ELISA for IgM, acute/convalescent IgG
Therapy: no antivirals; vitamin A, antibiotics for secondary bacterial infections
Vaccine: live attenuated vaccine (MMR), live virus

Measles or rubeola is an acute, highly infectious disease characterized by a maculopapular rash that often becomes confluent and blotchy. It is caused by the measles virus (morbillivirus), a member of the Paramyxoviridae family. In contrast with the influenza virus, the measles virion lacks neuraminidase.

Signs and symptoms. After contracting the virus, the incubation period lasts for two weeks prior to the development of a rash. Prior to the appearance of the rash, the patients suffer from a prodromal illness:

- Conjunctivitis
- Swelling of the eyelids
- Photophobia
- High fever (105°C)
- Hacking cough
- Rhinitis
- Malaise

A day or two before the rash develops, small bumps like grains of sand on an erythematous base of the buccal mucosa appear. They are called Koplik's spots and last for a day or two. The rash first appears in the face and neck, later spreading down the body. Within days, it takes on a darker color and can have a hemorrhagic appearance. The characteristic skin rash is due to damage inflicted by immune T lymphocytes on virus-infected endothelial cells.

Diagnosis. Clinical manifestations are sufficient for the diagnosis of measles.

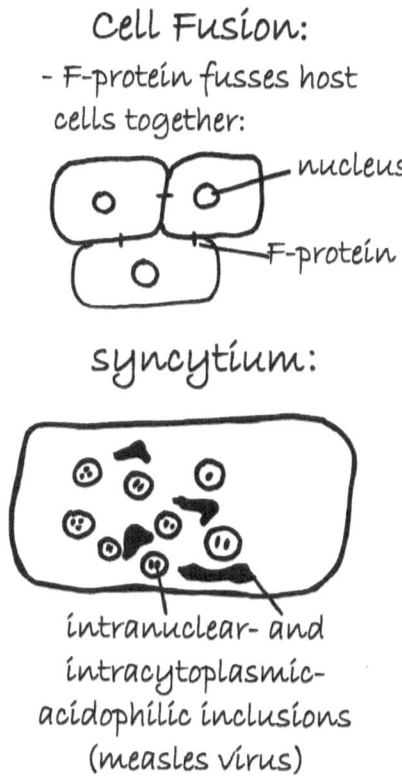

Cell Fusion:
- F-protein fusses host
cells together:
— nucleus
— F-protein

syncytium:

intranuclear- and
intracytoplasmic-
acidophilic inclusions
(measles virus)

Figure 5.4. Formation of syncytium

Sequelae. Measles is a distinct predilection for serious complications; among these are streptococcal or pneumococcal bronchopneumonia, encephalitis, otitis media, and mastoiditis.

Transmission. Measles is an extremely contagious disease that is spread by a respiratory route through nasopharyngeal secretions by air or by direct contact. Healthy carriers are unknown. The portal of entry is the mouth and nose. Measles is most communicable during the three to four days preceding the skin eruption. The virus lodges and multiplies in the mucosa of the respiratory, alimentary, and urinary tracts; conjunctival membranes; the endothelial cells of small blood vessels; and the lymphatics.

Treatment. Treatment for measles is primarily supportive. Low serum concentrations of vitamin A have been associated with severe measles, so vitamin A therapy should be considered. Antibiotic therapy is conducted for any of the bacterial complications that may occur.

Epidemiology. Humans are the only reservoir for measles in most parts of the world, although monkeys are also susceptible. Virtually an attack of measles produces a permanent immunity.

Prevention. The prevention of measles has been accomplished with a live measles vaccine. Ordinarily, the first dose is given as a part of the standard measles, mumps, and German measles vaccine at age of twelve to fifteen months. A second dose of measles vaccine is given on entry into school at an age of four to six years, a dose that can be given as early as one month after the initial one. All children should have their immunization record reviewed at eleven to twelve years of age.

Cultures. The virus has been grown in chick embryos, cultures of human, monkey, and dog kidney tissue, and in human cell lines. In cultures, multinucleate syncytial giant cells form by fusion of mononucleated ones, and others become spindle-shaped in the course of their degeneration. The measles virus is relatively unstable after it is released from cells. During the culture of the virus, the intracellular virus titer is ten or more times the extracellular.

Respiratory Syncytial Virus Infection

Table 5.5
Properties of Respiratory Syncytial Infection

Virion: spherical
Envelope: from cytoplasmic membrane
Capsid: helical
Genome: -ssRNA, 20 kb, 10 genes

Target cell type: respiratory epithelial cells, macrophages

Transmission: airborne—countertops or doorknobs

Diseases: "bad cold," bronchiolitis, and pneumonia in infants and children

Described in 1956 as the "chimpanzee coryza agent"

Respiratory syncytial virus (RSV), which causes lower respiratory tract infection, is a major cause of serious acute illness (bronchiolitis and viral pneumonia) in young children in both developing and developed countries. It is the most common cause of bronchiolitis. At the beginning of the illness, the virus replicates in the nasopharynx and spreads further through respiratory epithelium and alveolar macrophages.

The impact of the virus on adult population has been recognized as well. Those who appear to be at increased risk are adults with underlying cardiopulmonary disease, frail elderly individuals living in long-term care facilities or at home, and the severely immunocompromised.

Since RSV has a nonsegmented ssRNA genome, it does not have the capacity for reassortment of the genome as influenza virus does, undergoing antigenic shifts leading to influenza virus pandemics. Nevertheless, RSV has quite a mutable genome. This is due to its dependence on an RNA polymerase that lacks the capacity for RNA proofreading and editing. Because of this, it has genetic heterogeneity that is shaped by the selective pressures of the environment.

Signs and symptoms. The first signs and symptoms are the same as in mild upper respiratory infection. However, a typical symptom of RSV infection is nasal congestion with a discharge. Cough is common in 90%–97% of people. Occasionally, in 50% of patients, fever may reach 39°C–40°C. Lower respiratory tract involvement is common, with 30%–40% of patients having rales and wheezing on examination of the chest. Myalgias and malaise are more common in influenza than RSV infection. Croup is often caused by the parainfluenza virus and, less often, by a respiratory syncytial virus.

Incubation period. The incubation period of RSV respiratory disease is estimated to be five days.

Sequelae. During bronchiolitis, ciliated epithelial cells are destroyed, and bronchiolar epithelial necrosis is observed in the most severe cases. Pneumonitis may occur as the alveoli become filled with fluid. In the USA, 0.1% of infants that develop RSV lower respiratory infection die.

Transmission. RSV is highly contagious and can be spread through droplets containing the virus when someone coughs or sneezes. It also can live on surfaces (such as countertops or doorknobs) and on hands and clothing, so it can be easily spread when a person touches something contaminated.

Treatment. Most people do not need hospitalization and improve with supportive care.

Epidemiology. Each year in the United States, RSV causes lower respiratory tract illness (LRI) in 20%–30% of infants and leads to the hospitalization of approximately 1% of infants at a cost of three hundred to four hundred million dollars annually. These epidemics occur annually at regular, predictable intervals—mainly in the late fall, winter, and spring. The severity of the outbreaks varies.

Prevention. Breast-feeding reduces the risk of developing severe RSV infections in infants. In addition to maternal antibodies, other immune-modulating factors in human milk contribute to this protection.

Cultures. The virus grows in a variety of cell lines, including HEp-2, HeLa, and Vero cells. The typical syncytial cytopathic effect and viral replication vary significantly, depending upon the virus strain and condition of the cell culture.

Historical reference. Human RSV was recovered from a chimpanzee with respiratory symptoms in 1956. It was designated a chimpanzee coryza agent. The first report on the RVS infection was done in the 1960s. The infection was identified in adults with pneumonia.

Respiratory Infections with Human Parainfluenza Virus

Table 5.6
Properties of Human Parainfluenza Viruses (HPIV)

Alternative name: influenza D, hemadsorption viruses, croup-associated viruses
Size: 150–400 nm in diameter
Envelope: plasma membrane
Virion: spherical
Capsid: helical
Genome: 15 kb in length, contains 6–7 genes
Target cell type: epithelium of the respiratory tract
Transmission: inhalation of airborne virus and mucous membranes of the nose and throat
Diseases: croup (acute laryngotracheobronchitis), pharyngitis, bronchiolitis, pneumonia, otitis media, and laryngitis
Vaccine: none
Discovered in late 1950s

The human parainfluenza viruses (HPIV) replicate in the epithelium of the upper respiratory tract and spread from there to the lower respiratory tract. Genetically and antigenically, they divided into types 1 to 4, which belong to two genera:

• *Respirovirus* (HPIV-1 and HPIV-3)
• *Rubulavirus* (HPIV-2 and HPIV-4)

Human parainfluenza virus type 1 (HPIV-1) is the principal cause of laryngotracheobronchitis or croup. HPIV-1, 2, and 3 are collectively the second most common cause of respiratory infection in infants, young children, the immunocompromised, and the elderly, surpassed only by the respiratory syncytial virus. HPIV-4 is detected infrequently and is less likely to cause a severe disease. Table 5.7 contains the clinical conditions caused by the various HPIV types.

Two surface glycoproteins are found in all HPIV:

- The hemagglutinin-neuraminidase (HN; "spikes"), a tetramer involved in binding to the cellular receptors and destruction
- The fusion protein (F), a trimer that is responsible for induction of membrane fusion

Both of these HPIVs project through the lipid envelope and form the major antigenic targets for neutralizing antibodies. They also appear on the surface of infected cells. Their hydrophobic tails project into the virion, where they interact with the M protein to aid in virus assembly. The nucleocapsid core is composed of the following:

- Large RNA polymerase (L), a multifunctional protein that contains RNA-dependent RNA polymerase catalytic motifs
- The phosphoprotein (P), a protein required for L functioning (RNA-dependent RNA polymerase consisting of the P and L proteins)
- The nucleocapsid protein (NP), a protein that binds tightly to the viral genome, creating a template for the RNA-dependent RNA polymerase composed of the P and L proteins

Parainfluenza viruses are relatively unstable, and their activity falls off at freezing temperatures.

Signs and symptoms. Usual signs and symptoms may include any of the following:

- Cough
- Rapid, labored breathing

- Hoarseness and wheezing
- Redness of the eye
- Rhinitis
- Fever
- Anorexia
- Vomiting
- Diarrhea

Signs and symptoms are typically most severe in children aged three and younger because of their smaller airways. The viral shedding occurs for up to eleven days and even longer in immunocompromised hosts.

Table 5.7

Clinical Conditions Caused by the Various HPIV Types

Condition	Virus Type
Croup	HPIV-1, HPIV-2, HPIV-3
Bronchitis	HPIV-1, HPIV-3
Bronchopneumonia	HPIV-1, HPIV-3
Minor upper respiratory tract disease	HPIV-1, HPIV-3, HPIV-4
Pneumonia and bronchiolitis	HPIV-1, HPIV-3

Diagnosis. Virological diagnosis depends on three categories of tests:

- Rapid diagnosis tests (electron microscopy: examination of secretions; indirect immunofluorescence with antisera)
- Virus isolation (primarily monkey kidney and continuous diploid human fibroblasts)
- Serology (a wide variety of serological tests are available)

Incubation period. The incubation period for HPIVs generally ranges from two to seven days.

Sequelae. Most cases of croup are mild, and it is rare when the airway swells enough to interfere with breathing. Pneumonia is a rare but potentially a serious complication.

Transmission. HPIV are common community-acquired respiratory pathogens without ethnic, socioeconomic, gender, age, or geographic boundaries. It is airborne and highly contagious. HPIV remains infectious in airborne droplets for over an hour.

Treatment. If symptoms are severe, the infants should be admitted to hospital and nursed in plastic tents supplied with cool, moistened oxygen (croupette).

Epidemiology. Unlike influenza and respiratory syncytial viruses, the HPIVs do not cause large epidemics, though approximately eighteen thousand infants and children are hospitalized each year in the United States because of lower respiratory infection caused by HPIV-3. This virus causes yearly spring and summer epidemics in North America and Europe. Serologic surveys have shown that 90%–100% of children aged five years and older have antibodies to HPIV-3, and about 75% have antibodies to HPIV-1 and 2. Occasionally, outbreaks may occur in institutions where type 3 particularly spreads very effectively. Only a small number of studies have reported on the isolation or epidemiology of HPIV-4.

Prevention. No vaccine is currently available to protect against infection caused by any of the HPIVs.

Nipah Virus Encephalitis

Nipah is spilling over, and we are observing these small clusters of cases—and it's a matter of time that the right strain will come along and efficiently spread among people.

—Jonathan Epstein,
New York Times interview, 2012

Table 5.8
Properties of Nipah Virus

Size: varies, 120–500 nm

Capsid: filamentous

Envelope: plasma membrane

Genome: -ssRNA, nonsegmented, 18.2 kb

Reservoir: fruit bats

Transmission: direct contact with infected animals including humans; foodborne (ingestion of raw date palm sap)

Diseases: highly lethal febrile encephalitis in humans and a predominantly respiratory disease in pigs

First human case: Sungai Nipah, Negri Sembilan, Malaysia, 1998

Biosafety: level 4 pathogen

Nipah virus (NiV) is a newly recognized, emerging, highly pathogenic zoonotic virus that causes fatal encephalitis and, in some cases, respiratory disease in humans. At first, it begins with three to fourteen days of fever and a headache followed by drowsiness and disorientation. Then it ordinarily progresses to coma and death within twenty-four to forty-eight hours. In some cases, patients have a respiratory illness during the early part of their infections.

The disease was first described during 1998–1999 in Malaysia and Singapore when a large epidemic of fatal encephalitis occurred in humans, making 283 people sick and 109 dead. Many of those who survived suffered permanent and crippling neurological disorders. The reservoir of the disease is various flying foxes also known as fruit bats. They are messy eaters that eat fruits by masticating the pulp and then spitting out the juices and seeds. The presence of orchards on pig farms attracts fruit bats and exposes pigs to a contaminated fruit sap, causing mild infections in those farm animals. Via close contact with pigs, the NiV was passed to farmers, causing fatal encephalitis. The outbreak ended after more than one million pigs were culled and the movement of pigs was stopped. Since then, NiV has caused recurring outbreaks of fatal encephalitis in Bangladesh and sporadic outbreaks in India. The outbreaks in Bangladesh have demonstrated human-to-human and foodborne transmission of NiV, with a 75% mortality rate. In the most recent outbreak of NiV infection, from December 2009 to March 2010, in the Faridpur and Gopalganj districts of Bangladesh, there were seventeen cases and fifteen deaths, an 88% fatality rate.

NiV cannot only be transmitted to humans from animals but it also can be transmitted directly from human to human. Thus, in Bangladesh, half the reported cases between 2001 and 2008 were due to such transmissions. Drug investigations to date have been inconclusive, and the clinical usefulness of the available drugs is uncertain. Logically, the efforts to prevent transmission should first focus on decreasing bat access to date palm sap. Freshly collected date palm juice should also be boiled, and fruits should be thoroughly washed and peeled before consumption.

Family Rhabdoviridae

Rhabdoviruses infect mammals, birds, fish, insects, and plants. A large number of them have not been assigned to a genus. The animal rhabdoviruses replicate in the cytoplasm, but certain plant rhabdoviruses may replicate in the nucleus. The rhabdovirus of greatest medical interest is the rabies viruses, which belong to the genus *Lyssavirus*.

Rabies

Table 5.9
Properties of Rhabdoviridae

Virion: bullet shape, 200 nm × 75 nm

Envelope: from cytoplasmic membrane

Capsid: helical

Genome: -ssRNA, nonsegmented, 11–15 kb, 5 genes

Target cell type: neurons

Cytopathy: Sellers stain, "Negri bodies" (cytoplasmic inclusions in the infected nerve cells); eosinophilic (red) and basophilic (blue) granules in cytoplasm

Transmission: saliva (rabid animal bite); airborne in bat caves

Diseases: rabies

Therapy: immediate vaccination before symptoms appear

Vaccine: inactivated/killed virus

Rabies is an acute infection of the CNS that is almost always fatal. It causes severe progressive encephalitis, myelitis, and paralysis and is one of the world's leading causes of mortality. The glycoprotein (G) is known to be the only protein component of the viral envelope that mediates viral entry into the host cells.

Signs and symptoms. The disease always starts with malaise, and any of the following may also be present:

- Loss of appetite
- Headache
- Nausea
- Vomiting
- Sore throat
- Fever

(*rabidus* = *mad*)
- Bullet-shaped viruses

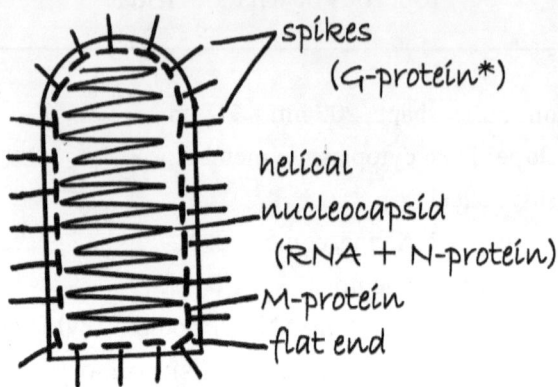

spikes
(G-protein*)

helical
nucleocapsid
(RNA + N-protein)
M-protein
flat end

*G (glyco-)- protein
(attachment protein):
- binds to a receptor on
the host cell surface

Figure 5.5. Architecture of Rhabdoviridae

The patient may show an increasing nervousness and apprehension. Usually, there is an abnormal sensation around the site of the infection. The act of swallowing water triggers an agonizing spasm of the throat muscles. Because of the patient's fear of water, the disease has been known as hydrophobia since antiquity. A patient may allow saliva to drool from his mouth simply to avoid swallowing and the associated painful spasms. After onset of symptoms, the infection progresses relentlessly. There are only three documented cases of symptomatic rabies of human patients who survived the disease. The last stage is followed by convulsive seizures and death. Paralysis may intervene before death but is not common.

Diagnosis. Postmortem diagnosis can be confirmed in man by demonstrating rabies antigen in the neurons of the hippocampus by both immunofluorescence and by histological Sellers staining that displays classical Negri bodies that are pathognomonic of rabies. These Negri bodies occur throughout the brain and spinal cord but are most frequently found in Ammon's horn of the hippocampus.

Incubation period. The incubation period in dogs ranges from three to eight weeks. The incubation period in man varies from two to sixteen weeks but may be as long as several years. It depends on the distance the virus has to move from its point of entry to the brain. It takes longer for the virus to cause symptoms if the individual had been bitten in the leg rather than in the face, and the incubation period is usually shorter in children than in adults.

Transmission. The rabies virus is ordinarily transmitted to man from the bite or scratch of an infected rabid animal. Rabid wild animals tend to be more prone to come into residential areas and act in atypical ways. They may bite even when unprovoked. Some individuals may come into contact with saliva on pets that have had an encounter with a rabid wild animal. The virus spreads from a wound contaminated with infected saliva through the sensory nerves to the CNS. It multiplies there and may spread through peripheral nerves to the salivary glands and other tissues. Rabies virus has a wide host range. All warm-blooded animals are susceptible. The virus is widely distributed in infected animals, having been detected in the nervous system, saliva, urine, lymph, milk, and blood. Recovery from an infection is rare, except in the vampire bats, in which the virus has become peculiarly adapted to the salivary glands. Airborne transmission may occur in caves where there are high densities of bats. The vampire bats may transmit the virus for months without themselves ever showing any signs of disease. Vampire bats kill thousands of cattle each year in Latin America while speleologists occasionally die following inhalation of the aerosols created by the secretions of insectivorous bats roosting in caves. Biting behavior is not a consequence of a rabies-induced neurologic disease in humans, and human-to-human transmission does not occur.

Rabies virus-infected cells:

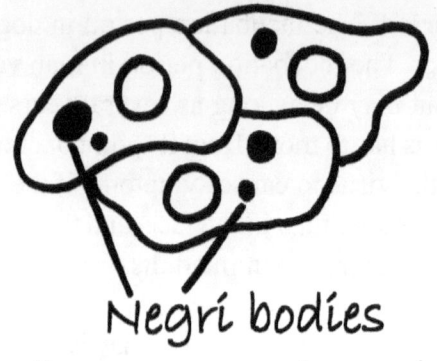

Negri bodies (intra cytoplasmic-acidophilic inclusions)

Figure 5.6. Negri bodies

Treatment. Active immunization with inactivated rabies vaccine should be administered shortly after individual had been bitten by an animal without confirmation of the rabies infection.

Epidemiology. In the USA, raccoons, skunks, foxes, and bats are the most important reservoirs of rabies; half the cases in humans have been related to the bites of bats. Man is an accidental host and is not a reservoir of rabies infection. With few exceptions such as in Australia, New Zealand, Hawaii, and Antarctica, rabies occurs throughout the world especially in India, Africa, and parts of Europe. Jackals and mongooses are the most important carriers of the infection to man in India and South Africa. Rabies affects more than fifty thousand people worldwide each year. In the USA, several thousand cases of animal rabies are reported annually—although human rabies is rare, fewer than five cases per year. Individuals subjected to high risk are veterinarians, mailmen, and medical students working with stray dogs in areas where canine vaccination is not compulsory.

Prevention. Rabies is best controlled by destroying stray dogs in cities and by compulsory vaccinations of all others. During outbreaks and for at least six months after each reported case, all dogs should be muzzled. In areas where vampire bats or foxes transmit rabies, prophylactic vaccination of cattle should be carried out.

Cultures. The virus is sampled from patient's saliva taken from under the tongue from submaxillary salivary gland. Bacteria in the sample are inactivated by penicillin and streptomycin. Saliva is then inoculated into mice (intracerebrally) or hamsters (intramuscularly). Inoculated mice ordinarily develop flaccid paralysis of the legs and then die. The virus also may be propagated in chick embryos or in tissue cultures prepared from mouse or chick embryos.

Historical reference. For centuries, the saliva of a rabid dog was thought to be the source of rabies infection, but it was only in 1804 that a German scientist, Georg Gottfried Zinke, succeeded in transmitting rabies from it. In 1884, long before the recognition of the nature of viruses, Louis Pasteur developed the world's first man-made viral vaccine from dessicated spinal cords of rabies-infected rabbits. On July 6, 1885, his dramatic demonstration of its efficacy in saving the life of a peasant boy, Joseph Meister, who had been bitten fourteen times by a rabid dog, heralded a new era in medicine.

Family Bunyaviridae

The family Bunyaviridae contains more than three hundred viruses, most of them being arthropod borne. Members of this family have many common characteristics: they are enveloped and amorphous (90–110 nm in diameter), with a trisegmented negative-stranded RNA genome, with replication occurring in the cytoplasm and budding taking place in the Golgi complex. The natural hosts for Bunyaviridae are a wide variety of arthropods and mammals. Transmission usually occurs via vectors such as ticks and mosquitoes or contact with infected animals or humans.

The Bunyaviridae family is divided into five different genera:

- *Phlebovirus*
- *Nairovirus*
- *Hantavirus*
- *Orthobunyavirus*
- *Tospovirus*

Many of them are serious human pathogens causing encephalitis or hemorrhagic fever. There are no vaccines currently available for any of them. Due to the large size of the virus family, the effects of these viruses on host organisms vary greatly. Usually, once contracted, the virus replicates in specific target organs. The types of affected organs and the severity of the disease depend on the type of virus causing the infection.

California and La Crosse Encephalitis

Table 5.10
Properties of genus *Bunyavirus*

Virion: amorphous, ~100 nm
Envelope: from Golgi membrane system
Capsid: helical
Genome: -ssRNA, 12–23 kb
Sentinel host: humans, domestic animals
Target cell type: endothelial cells
Transmission: mosquito-borne
Vector: mosquitoes, ticks
Reservoir: chipmunks, squirrels, rabbits, and hares
Diseases: California encephalitis, La Crosse encephalitis
Vaccine: none

California encephalitides are caused mostly by the La Crosse virus transmitted by *Aedes triseriatus*. The La Crosse virus is a member of the genus *Bunyavirus*. California encephalitis, La Crosse encephalitis, and Rift Valley fever (an African virus of genus *Phlebovirus*), are all collectively called arboviral encephalitis. They are all caused by different viruses, though the clinical manifestations of the diseases are very similar to each other. Viremia begins with the reticuloendothelial system, especially at the liver, spleen, and lymph nodes. Then it spreads to the CNS in the site of endothelial cells of the cerebral capillary system or the choroid plexus. It is rare when the viral infection moves further to the tissue of the brain.

Signs and symptoms. Commonly, when infected adults become carriers of the disease, their infection is asymptomatic. In children, the virus causes an onset of nonspecific symptoms such as chills, fever, nausea, vomiting, headache, and abdominal pain. It is characterized by drowsiness, lack of mental alertness, and orientation and paralysis. A total of 10% of patients develop coma. Seizures occur in 50% of children. Approximately 20% recurrent, unprovoked seizures occur even after the illness has passed. The total duration of an illness rarely exceeds ten to fourteen days.

In adults, an infection is often asymptomatic or causes benign febrile illness or aseptic meningitis.

Incubation period. The incubation period of California encephalitis is usually three to seven days.

Sequelae. Mortality is low (0.3%), but 10% of patients suffer neurological sequelae: recurring seizures and behavioral problems.

Transmission. The principal vector of La Crosse is *Aedes triseriatus*. It breeds in tree holes, but abandoned tires filled with rainwater constitute an important breeding area for this as well as for other mosquito species that could serve as a potential vector close to human habitation.

Epidemiology. The highest incidence of encephalitides in the USA, seventy-five cases annually, is in the Midwestern States, usually in late summer or early fall. The woodland areas are associated with an increased risk of infection. La Crosse encephalitis has been reported in twenty-eight states.

Treatment. There is no treatment against the California encephalitis virus. Treatment is given only to manage the symptoms. Supportive treatment includes mechanical ventilation and the use of steroids to reduce brain inflammation. Sometimes, sedatives are used to control irritability or restlessness. To reduce fever and headache, acetaminophen is used, and to prevent seizures, anticonvulsants are used.

Prevention. No vaccine exists for the virus; control measures have involved control of the mosquito vector.

Historical reference. The California encephalitis virus was first isolated in 1943 from mosquitoes collected in Kern County, California. Two years later, three human cases of an infection leading to encephalitis were attributed to this new virus. Since then, most cases have been associated with the La Crosse virus that had been isolated from the brain of a four-year-old boy who died of the infection in La Crosse County, Wisconsin. These viruses now are classified within the genus *Bunyavirus* of the family Bunyaviridae.

Hantavirus Infections

Hantavirus infections are severe infections that manifest either as hemorrhagic fever renal syndrome (HFRS) or hantavirus cardiopulmonary syndrome (HPS), with many similar symptoms. HPS was formally known as Four Corners diseases (see epidemiology). In 1993, an epidemic was called Sin Nombre virus. Hemorrhagic fever with renal syndrome was formally known as Korean hemorrhagic fever. It is a manifestation of a disease caused by closely related viruses.

Table 5.11
Properties of Hantavirus

Virion: amorphous, 100 nm

Envelope: from Golgi membrane system

Capsid: three nucleocapsids, helical

Genome: -ssRNA, trisegmented,

Target cell type: endothelial cells

Transmission: aerosolized rodent urine or feces

Reservoir: rodents of the orders Murinae, Arvicolinae, and Sigmodontinae; mice: *Peromyscus maniculatus* (in the United States), *Apodemus agrarius* (in Korea), and *Apodemus flavicollis* (in Eastern Europe and China); rats: *Rattus norvegicus* (in Korea); humans are dead-end hosts

Diseases: hemorrhagic fever

Vaccine: none

Causative agent. Viruses of Hantavirus genus are the causative agents of HPS and HFRS. The genus *Hantavirus* of the Bunyaviridae family was named after the Hantan River in South Korea. After the virus gets into the lungs through inhalation, it immediately invades capillaries. The immune mechanisms play a significant role in the pathogenesis. Capillary leakage is caused by following factors:

- Early T cell activation
- Unusual increase of neutrophils, monocytes, B cells
- Increased levels of cytokines in circulation
- Activation of kinin system along with classical and alternative complement systems
- Formation of immune complexes that damage the vascular endothelium

Because of the early appearance of IgM and IgE antibody complexes, some researchers suggest that HFRS is an allergic disease.

Signs and symptoms. A hantavirus infection is rare but deadly. Early symptoms of HPS include malaise; chills; fever; headache; dizziness; myalgia in the thighs, hips, and back; nausea; diarrhea; and vomiting or abdominal pain; four to ten days after those symptoms, coughing, tachycardia, and tachypnea appear. This can lead to cardiovascular shock and death.

The symptoms of HFRS manifest in five stages:

- The febrile stage is similar to the early symptoms of HPS.
- The hypotensive stage is characterized by a two-day duration of dyspnea and tachycardia.
- The oliguric stage manifests as an onset of renal failure and proteinuria, an excess of serum proteins in the urine that lasts for three days or a week.
- The diuretic stage is characterized by polyuria (3–6 L per day) that lasts for several days up to weeks.
- The convalescent stage is a period when conditions seem to improve and patient is in recovery.

Incubation period. The incubation period varies from four to forty-two days.

Sequelae. Usual complications are kidney, lung, and heart failure and death. HPS fatality rate may reach 60%. The mortality rate for the North American HPS is over 30%. HFRS mortality and morbidity rates vary, depending on the strand of the virus; it can be as low as 5% or as high as 15%. In children and adolescents younger than fifteen years old, the disease is mild and often subclinical.

Diagnoses. Blood tests reveal if there are antibodies against hantavirus present.

Transmission. People become infected if either in direct contact with droppings, urine, or saliva of mice, especially deer mice and rats, or inhalation of those aerosolized excretions. The viruses do not cause serious disease in their rodent hosts like they do in humans. This disease does not transmit from person to person.

Epidemiology. Viruses related to hantaviruses have been isolated from all over the world, including the United States. HPS is more common in the rural areas of the Western United States during the spring and summer months. It also occurs in Canada and South America. Unlike other forms of HPS and HFTS, the South American disease is a milder variety of the HPS infection that could be transmitted from person to person. HFRS occurs mainly in Europe and Asia. Severe cases of the disease appear in China, Japan, and Singapore, 100,000–250,000 cases annually. Mild forms of the disease occur in Scandinavian countries.

Treatment. One has to fight hantavirus on one's own since there is no antiviral treatment. However, immediate hospitalization is required. Supportive therapy is often necessary such as maintaining the oxygen level either by mechanical ventilation or intubation (placing tubes in the nose, mouth, or trachea) along with fluid replacement. In extremely severe cases, extracorporeal membrane oxygenation, the pumping of a patient's blood through a machine that removes carbon dioxide and adds oxygen, is necessary. To treat kidney-related problems, ribavirin may be used. Unfortunately, this medication may cause serious birth defects and even fetal death if used during pregnancy.

Prevention. To prevent an infection, one should avoid rodent dens. A mouse can squeeze through a very small hole. Therefore, those holes should be sealed either with cement, metal flashing, or wire screening. There should be no mice access to food or trash. To prevent mice nesting, keep junk away from the house's foundation. When spring-loaded traps are used, dead animals and areas where mice had been should be wet with household bleach or alcohol. Mice droppings and nests should be sprayed with 10% bleach solution or disinfectant.

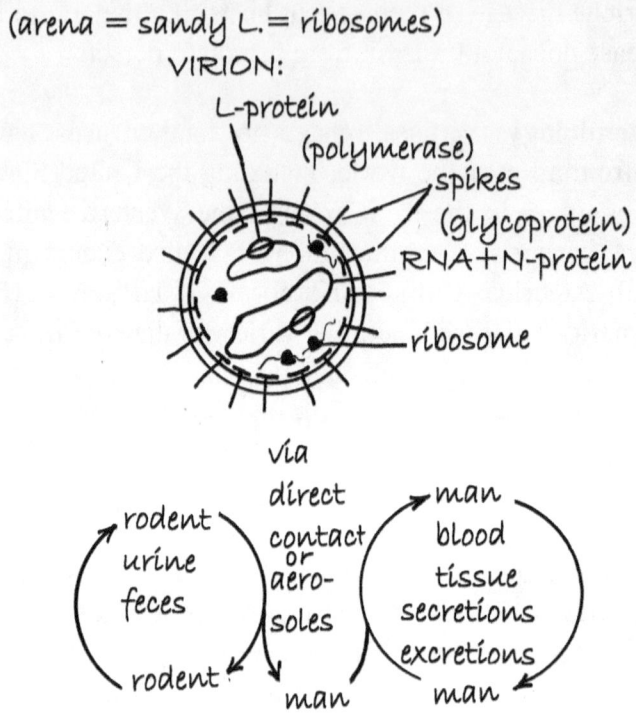

Figure 5.7. Architecture and transmission of Arenaviridae

This will prevent infected dust from being stirred up into the air. After the area is mopped with disinfectant, rubber gloves and a wet towel should be used to pick up any residue. Cleaning material and used gloves should be disposed in a plastic bag. A vacuum should not be used before areas are first decontaminated.

Historical reference. Between 1913 and 1930, HFRS was recognized by Soviet scientists who described the disease in the eastern part of the Soviet Union. During the Korean War, thousands of the United Nation soldiers became sick with what they called Korean hemorrhagic fever. It took twenty-five years to identify the cause of the disease. The causative agent, the Hantaan virus (HTNV), was isolated in 1970s in South Korea by Ho Wang Lee and his colleagues.

In 1993, there was an epidemic of HPS in the Four Corners region of the USA: southwestern corner of Colorado, northwestern corner of

New Mexico, northeastern corner of Arizona, and southeastern corner of Utah. A few weeks later, a deer mouse, *Peromyscus maniculatus,* was identified by Terry Yates, a professor of the University of New Mexico, as a host harboring several viruses of the *Hantavirus* genus that caused this outbreak.

Family Arenaviridae

Table 5.12
Properties of Arenaviridae

Size: 100 nm

Envelope: from endoplasmic reticulum

Capsid: undefined morphology, 11 kb

Genome: –ssRNA, two segments: L(arge) and S(mall)

Sentinel host: humans

Target cell type: numerous cell types (monocytes, dendritic cells, fibroblastic reticular cells, etc.)

Transmission: respiratory—aerosolized rodent urine or feces

Reservoir: rodents

Diseases: hemorrhagic fever, LCM, Machupo, etc.

Arenaviridae share many features with the hantaviruses since they both coevolved with rodents. Like hantaviruses, they establish a persistent infection in a single rodent host, transmitted to humans by aerosolized rodent urine or feces. At least eight arenaviruses are known to cause human disease. Because of their association with a single rodent species, their geographic range is restricted to that of their host. The exceptions are rodents that had been distributed by humans such as the house mouse and the urban rat.

Table 5.13
Arenaviruses—Diseases and Geography

Virus	Vector	Diseases	Distribution
Lymphocytic choriomeningitis virus	house mouse	lymphocytic choriomeningitis	worldwide
Lassa virus	natal multimammate	Lassa fever	West Africa
Junin virus	drylands vesper mouse	Argentine hemorrhagic fever	Argentina
Machupo virus	large vesper mouse	Bolivian hemorrhagic fever	Bolivia
Guanarito virus	short-tailed cane mouse	Venezuelan hemorrhagic fever	Venezuela
Sabiá virus	unknown	Brazilian hemorrhagic fever	Brazil
Flexal virus	rice rat	influenza-like illness	Brazil
Whitewater Arroyo virus	wood rat	hemorrhagic fever	Southwestern USA

Family Filoviridae

The Marburg virus (MARV) and the Ebola virus (EBOV) genera are members of the family Filoviridae, best known as causative agents of acute hemorrhagic fevers. They are responsible for mortality rates of up to 88% in outbreaks involving hundreds of people.

Their genome sequences suggest that they are most closely related to the pneumoviruses, and they are assumed to replicate in a manner similar to that of the rhabdoviruses and paramyxoviruses.

Ebola Hemorrhagic Fever

Table 5.14
Properties of Ebola Virus

Size: ~800–1000 nm × 80 nm

Virion: filament

Envelope: from cytoplasmic membrane

Capsid: helical

Genome: -ssRNA, 19 kb, 7 genes

Target cell type: numerous cell types (monocytes, dendritic cells, fibroblastic reticular cells, etc.)

Transmission: contact with or eating infected wildlife, especially gorillas

Diseases: Ebola hemorrhagic fever

Reservoir: various bats

Biosafety: level 4

First human case: Yambuku region, Zaire (Democratic Republic of Congo), 1976

Vaccine: none

Ebola hemorrhagic fever is a severe febrile hemorrhagic disease caused by the Ebola virus (EBOV) of the Filoviridae family. The virus causing Ebola hemorrhagic fever was named after the Congo River in Africa, which is pronounced *Ebola* in French. The virus was first identified in 1976.

Causative agent. The virus is a member of a family of filamentous RNA viruses called Filoviridae. There are five identified subtypes of Ebola viruses, four of which cause diseases in humans: Ebola-Zaire, Ebola-Sudan, Ebola–Ivory Coast, and Ebola-Bundibugyo. The fifth, Ebola-Reston, does not cause any signs and symptoms in humans but kills nonhuman primates and pigs.

Signs and symptoms. Ebola hemorrhagic fever is an acute disease in humans and nonhuman primates such as monkeys, gorillas, and chimpanzees. There is no carrier state. The onset of the illness is abrupt and is characterized by extremely high fever, headache, arthralgia, myalgia, malaise, and sore throat, followed by diarrhea, vomiting, stomach pain, and loss of weight. In some patients, there are rashes, red eyes, hiccups, and severe skin and internal organ hemorrhage. The Ebola HF virus interferes with the immune system's ability to mount a defense. The patients who die usually do not develop a significant immune response to the disease. Why some people die while others are capable of surviving is not understood.

Filoviridae

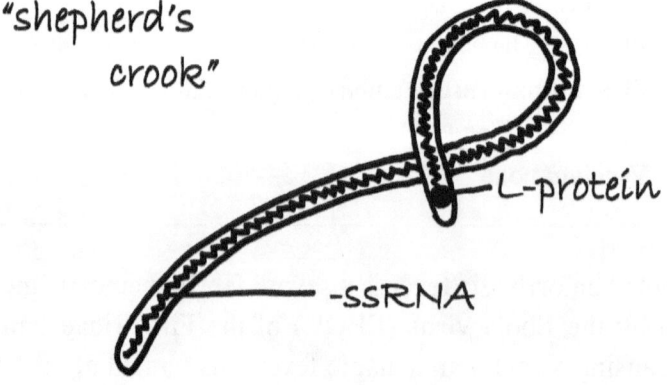

Figure 5.8. Architecture of Filoviridae

Incubation period. The incubation period ranges from two to twenty-one days.

Sequelae. For those who survive Ebola HF, the recovery is a very slow process, taking months to gain strength and weight. People may experience hair loss, hepatitis, sensory change, and eye and testicular inflammation.

Diagnoses. Clinical diagnosis is difficult because signs and symptoms are nonspecific to the virus. However, if anyone has the constellation of symptoms and is suspected to have Ebola HF infection, then the patient has to be isolated from others to avoid an outbreak of this often fatal disease. Within three days after the onset of symptoms, ELISA testing, PCR, and virus isolation can be used for diagnostic purposes. Later in the course of the disease, a person can be tested for IgM and IgG antibodies.

Transmission. Nosocomial transmission often occurs during outbreaks of Ebola HF infections. Beside health workers, people can become infected through contact with infected friends and family members while taking care of them. The disease is extremely infectious but not extremely contagious, meaning it takes an extremely small amount of viruses to cause illness. It is not extremely contagious because the transmission occurs through contact with infected blood or secretions; it is not airborne.

Epidemiology. The natural reservoir of infection remains unknown. Perhaps, the virus is animal-borne (zoonotic), occurring in an animal host native to Africa.

It is likely that a subtype of Ebola-Reston is associated with a similar subtype in the Philippines. This virus was isolated from monkeys imported from Philippines to the USA and Italy. Its virus caused severe diseases and death in those imported animals. Nonhuman primates are even more sensitive to the Ebola HF virus than humans. Several researchers, who worked with the animals, became infected but did not appear clinically ill. Ebola HF had appeared in sporadic outbreaks in native continents. However, this year, 2014, Ebola outbreaks became epidemic. WHO reports 4,033 people have died so far, with 8,399 suspected cases. The disease became widely spread in Guinea, Liberia, and Sierra Leone. The rates of transmission of Ebola in those countries are intense. So far, countries with localized infections include Nigeria, Senegal, Spain, and the USA.

Treatment. Since there is no standard treatment for the Ebola HF, patients must receive supportive therapy. This includes balancing the patient's fluid and electrolyte levels, maintaining oxygen status, replacing blood loss, and treating every secondary infection that develops.

Prevention. It is challenging to prevent Ebola HF since the identity and natural reservoir of the infection is unknown. Health-care providers should be able to recognize a case of Ebola HF should one appear and be ready to employ practical viral hemorrhagic fever isolation precautions or barrier nursing techniques such as the use of protective clothing (face shields, double gloves, gowns, goggles, leg and shoe coverings) plus complete equipment sterilization. More research in identifying the natural reservoir of the Ebola HF virus and routes of its transmission must be acquired to prevent future outbreaks.

Historical reference. In 1976, the disease appeared sporadically in Yambuku, Democratic Republic of the Congo (DRC, formally Zaire). A total of 318 people were infected, 280 of whom died. It was spread by close personal contact and by the use of contaminated needles and syringes in hospitals and clinics. In the same year, 248 cases of the infection were identified in Sudan (Nzara, Maridi, and surrounding areas), where 151 people died. The disease was associated with hospitals in which many personal workers were infected. In England, a laboratory researcher was accidentally stuck with a needle but survived the infection. On October 12, 2014, a nurse at Texas Presbyterian Hospital who provided care for the Ebola patient became the first person infected with Ebola on US soil.

Table 5.15
Major Outbreaks of Ebola Hemorrhagic Fever

Location	Year	Number of Infected Individuals	Fatality Cases	Transmission
Sudan	1979	34	22	
Gabon	1994	52	51	
DRC	1995	315	250	The infection spread from families and hospitals had been traced to one patient who worked in the forest adjoining the city.
Gabon	1996–1997	97	66	The infection was spread by hunters who butchered and ate chimpanzees.
Uganda	2000–2001	425	224	
DRC	2002–2003	178	157	
DRC	2007	264	187	
Uganda	Dec 2007–Jan 2008	149	37	
Liberia	as of October 8, 2014	4076	2316	
Sierra Lione	as of October 8, 2014	2950	930	
Guinea	as of October 8, 2014	1350	778	

Nigeria	as of October 8, 2014	20	8	
Senegal	as of October 8, 2014	1	0	The infection originated in Guinea.
Spain	as of October 8, 2014	1	0	
USA	as of October 14, 2014	2	1	In one case, patient-nurse transmission on the US soil.

Marburg Hemorrhagic Fever

Table 5.16
Properties of Marburg Hemorrhagic Fever Virus

Size: ~800 nm × 80 nm
Virion: filament
Envelope: from cytoplasmic membrane
Capsid: helical
Genome: 19 kb, seven genes
Target cell type: numerous cell types (monocytes, dendritic cells, fibroblastic reticular cells, etc.)
Transmission: unknown
Diseases: Marburg hemorrhagic fever
Vaccine: none

Marburg hemorrhagic fever is a severe type of hemorrhagic fever caused by the Marburg virus of the Filoviridae family. Marburg hemorrhagic fever (HF) is also referred as Marburg virus disease.

Previously, it had been known as green monkey disease due to its origin of discovery.

Causative agent. The causative agent is a helical, enveloped, nonsegmented negative-stranded RNA virus called Lake Victoria Marburgvirus, belonging to the family Filoviridae. Recognition of the Marburg HF virus led to the creation of this new virus family that now also includes Ebola HF viruses. The virus is very similar in its structure to Ebola HF viruses, though it elicits different antibodies in the host body.

Signs and symptoms. The onset of the disease is marked by chills, fevers, headache, and myalgia. After the first symptoms, usually on the fifth day, a maculopapular rash appears most prominently on the chest, back, and stomach, followed by nausea, a sore throat, chest pain, and diarrhea. Symptoms become increasingly severe and may include jaundice, severe weight loss, delirium, inflammation of the pancreas, liver failure, massive hemorrhaging, and multiple organ dysfunction.

Incubation period. The onset of the disease is sudden, in about five to ten days after the infection takes place.

Sequelae. Recovery from Marburg HF may be prolonged and accompanied by recurrent hepatitis, orchitis, transverse myelitis, uveitis, and parotitis.

Diagnoses. If only a single case is involved, clinical diagnosis are difficult because signs and symptoms are similar to malaria, typhoid fever, and Ebola HF. In addition to PCR and virus isolation, the same serological testing is usually done as in cases with Ebola HF.

Transmission. The reservoir and how an animal host transmits Marburg HF virus to humans remain unknown. Recently, the African fruit bat, *Rousettus aegyptiacus*, had been strongly suspected to be a reservoir of the infection.

Infected people, who handled infected monkeys, had been in contact with their fluids or cell cultures. As with Ebola HF, nosocomial transmission is common. Droplets of body fluids of infected people (contaminated with those fluids), equipment, and other objects are highly suspected as sources of the disease.

Epidemiology. Marburg HF is a very rare human disease. It appears in sporadic outbreaks throughout Africa, often in males working in mines and their family members and health-care workers who had been in contact with infected miners.

Treatment. There is no specific treatment for Marburg HF. The same supportive therapy is administrated as in cases with Ebola HF.

Prevention. Preventive measures have not yet been established due to the limited knowledge of the disease. If a patient is suspected to have Marburg HF, barrier nursing techniques should be used to prevent direct physical contact with the patient. It is important to increase awareness among health-care providers about the signs and symptoms that suggest Marburg HF in patients.

Historical reference. The first simultaneous outbreak occurred in 1967 in Marburg and Frankfurt, Germany, and Belgrade, Yugoslavia (now Serbia), and in the laboratories handling green monkeys, *Cercopithecus aethiops*. They had been imported from Uganda for research purposes and for the preparation of polio vaccine; thirty-one people became infected, seven died. Other larger outbreaks occurred as follows:

- In the DRC, in 1988–2000, young men working in the gold mine in Durba were infected, and the infection spread to the neighboring villages; of 154 people infected, 128 died.
- In Angola, in 2004–2005, an outbreak begun in the Uíge Province, infecting 252 people, killing 227.
- Additionally, there were single-case outbreaks during 1975–2008 in South Africa, Kenya, Uganda, the USA, and the Netherlands.

CHAPTER VI

Double-Stranded RNA Viruses

Family Reoviridae

Table 6.1
Properties of Reoviridae

Size: 70–95 nm
Envelope: nonenveloped
Capsid: icosahedral, 92 capsomers
Genome: dsRNA, 10–12 segments, 20–30 kb
Sentinel hosts: humans and domestic animals
Reservoir: vertebrates
Vector: insects (mosquitoes, culicoides, and ticks)
Diseases: gastroenteritis and infantile diarrhea

Reoviridae is the largest and most diverse family of dsRNA viruses. It includes twelve established genera with over 150 species. These are medium-sized viruses that replicate in cytoplasm. The hosts of these viruses include plants, vertebrates, insects, and fungi. The viruses of this family, with the exception of the *Cytoplasmic polyhedrosis* virus, consist of an inner core that is surrounded by a few layers of protein that encapsidates nine to twelve segments of dsRNA and the enzymes involved in transcription. The viruses have similar morphologies of the innermost capsid shells but a different sequence homology among component proteins. The outer capsid shell appears to play an important role in maintaining the stability of the thin innermost capsid with the dsRNA genome. Reoviridae are ubiquitous in nature.

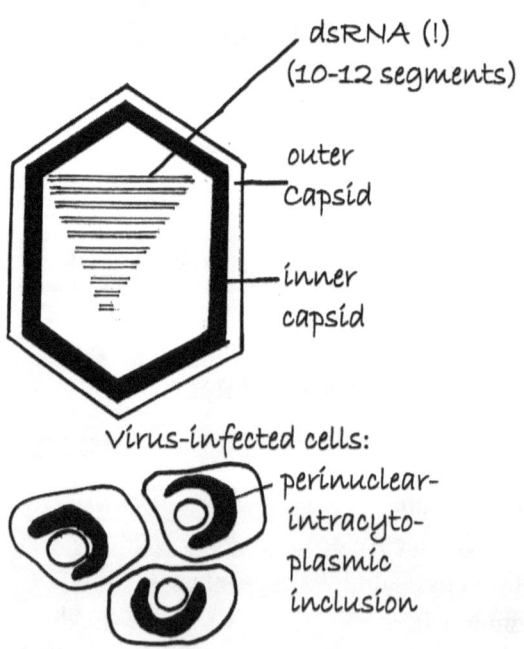

Figure 6.1. Architecture of Reoviridae

They can affect the gastrointestinal system and respiratory tract. Infections cause epidemic gastroenteritis and infantile diarrhea.

Family Rotaviruses

Table 6.2
Properties of Rotaviruses

Size: 70 nm

Capsid: icosahedral

Envelope: mature viruses do not possess envelope

Composition: three protein shells, an outer capsid, an inner capsid, and an internal core

Genome: 11 genome segments (dsRNA), each segment is a gene;

18,555 nucleotides in total

Sentinel host: humans, domestic animals

Target cell type: the mature epithelial cells of the small intestine, viremia is possible; respiratory tract, liver, kidney

Transmission: fecal-oral contact, via contact with contaminated hands, surfaces, and objects

Diseases: diarrhea, primarily in newborns and the young children

Vaccine: attenuated virus

Rotaviruses are the most common cause of viral gastroenteritis in infants and young children. More than 90% of children in the USA have been infected by the age of three. In the USA, the infection results in twenty to seventy childhood deaths annually. Worldwide, each year, rotavirus causes ~114 million episodes of gastroenteritis requiring home care and 2.4 million hospitalizations in children under five years of age, killing 1 in 205. The rotavirus causes approximately 39% of childhood diarrhea hospitalizations worldwide. After a first natural infection, infants and young children are protected against subsequent symptomatic disease.

In temperate climates, rotavirus disease occurs during the cooler months. Acquired immunity makes rotavirus infections much less common in adults. The incubation period is two to three days. The infection manifests as a low-grade fever, diarrhea, and vomiting and subsides in about one week. Dehydration and electrolyte disturbances are the major sequelae of rotavirus infection. Diagnosis is achieved by several types of commercially available tests based on enzyme immunoassays. Treatment is limited to oral rehydration.

Human rotaviruses exhibit colossal diversity, giving rise to various strains. Most human rotaviruses belong to serogroups A, B, and C. Group A rotaviruses are the most important from a public health standpoint. The majority of mothers have rotavirus antibody from previous infection that is passed transplacentally, protecting the neonate, who will have an asymptomatic or mild disease. Two oral attenuated rotavirus vaccines are used since 2006:

- The pentavalent bovine-human reassortant vaccine (RotaTeq)
- The monovalent human rotavirus vaccine (Rotarix)

They has been used in ~100 countries worldwide, proving to be safe and having a high efficacy profile in Western industrialized countries and in Latin America. More new rotavirus vaccines are now in development.

Hepatitis D

Hepatitis D, an acute infection of the liver caused by the hepatitis D virus (HDV), is often referred as delta hepatitis. HDV is a small partially double-stranded, circular, enveloped RNA virus, structurally unrelated to HAV, HBV, and HCV. It is the smallest RNA virus identified to date among the animal viruses. In order to propagate, the HDV requires the presence of HBV, which encodes the coat protein for HDV, putting it in a category of subviral satellite viruses.

Table 6.3
Properties of Hepatitis D Virus

Alternative name: "delta" hepatitis from subviral satellite viruses

Size: 35–37 nm spherical particle enveloped by a lipoprotein coat derived from HBsAg

Envelope: requires hepatitis B virus as a helper to acquire coat proteins

Genome: 1.7 kb, dsRNA

Target cell type: hepatocytes

Transmission: coinfection with Hepatitis B, superinfection of hepatitis B carrier

Diseases: hepatitis D, cirrhosis, fulminant hepatitis

Complications: cirrhosis of liver, hepatocellular carcinoma, and a fulminant hepatic failure

Vaccine: none

Discovered: in 1977 by Mario Rizzetto

There are three known genotypes:

- Genotype 1 (distributed worldwide)
- Genotype 2 (in Taiwan, Japan, and Northern Asia)
- Genotype 3 (in South America)

The incubation period is about twenty-one to forty-five days. Hepatitis D is clinically indistinguishable from other forms of viral hepatitis; symptoms include fever, malaise, headache, dark urine, vomiting, and jaundice. The presence of antibodies directed against HDAg is an indication of an HDV infection. The coinfection or superinfection with hepatitis D leads to highest mortality rates of all hepatitis infections, leading to a greater likelihood of an acute infection and the rapid progression of cirrhosis of the liver, hepatocellular carcinoma, and a fulminant hepatic failure of 80%–90%.

Transmission of HDV occurs the same way as transmission of HBV: parenterally, through blood transfusion, sharing needles for drugs, tattooing, or piercing. Sexual transmission of hepatitis D is less efficient than with HBV.

Transmission of HDV may occur in two ways:

- Via simultaneous with HV (coinfection)
- Via an infection previously infected with a HBV individual (superinfection)

Epidemiology. HDV is more common in adults than in children. About fifteen million people are infected worldwide. Approximately 10%–20% of all chronic HBV carriers are infected with HDV. The most affected areas are Southern Italy, North Africa, the Middle East, the Amazon Basin, and the American South Pacific islands.

Treatment. There is no effective treatment at this time. Many of the medications used for treating hepatitis B are not useful in treatment of hepatitis D. Some patient might require alpha interferon treatment. A liver transplant at the end stage of acute infection may be effective.

Prevention. People with an HBV infection are susceptible to hepatitis D. The use of condoms may reduce but not eliminate the transmission of hepatitis D. Because the HDV envelope contains HBsAg, the HBV vaccine also protects against HDV. Hepatitis B vaccine for noncarriers of hepatitis B is recommended.

Cultures. There is no line cell susceptible to a hepatitis D infection.

Historical reference. In 1970s, Turin, Italy, researchers detected and described the delta antigen from carriers of Hepatitis B. At first, the delta antigen was thought to be a component of the HBV.

Collaboration of Italian and American scientists led to experiments with chimpanzees, which demonstrated that the delta antigen was not a component but a separate virus that requires HBV for its propagation. It was named the hepatitis D virus.

BIBLIOGRAPHY

Aguilar, P. V., A. P. Adams, E. Wang, W. Kang, A. S. Carrara, M. Anishchenko, I. Frolov, and S. C. Weaver. "Structural and Nonstructural Protein Genome Regions of Eastern Equine Encephalitis Virus Are Determinants of Interferon Sensitivity and Murine Virulence." *Journal of Virology* 82 (2008): 4920–4930.

Aguilar, P. V., L. W. Leung, E. Wang, S. C. Weaver, and C. F. Basler. "A Five-Amino-Acid Deletion of the Eastern Equine Encephalitis Virus Capsid Protein Attenuates Replication in Mammalian Systems but Not in Mosquito Cells." *Journal of Virology* 82 (2008): 6972–6983.

Aguilar, P. V., S. Paessler, A. S. Carrara, S. Baron, J. Poast, E. Wang, A. C. Moncayo, M. Anishchenko, D. Watt, R. B. Tesh, and S. C. Weaver. "Variation in Interferon Sensitivity and Induction among Strains of Eastern Equine Encephalitis Virus." *Journal of Virology* 79 (2005): 11300–11310.

American Academy of Pediatrics. "Parainfluenza Viral Infections." In *Red Book: 2009 Report of the Committee on Infectious Diseases*. 28th ed., edited by L. K. Pickering, C. J. Baker, D. W. Kimberlin, and S. S. Long. Elk Grove Village, Illinois, 2009: 485–487.

Atasheva, S., N. Garmashova, I. Frolov, and E. Frolova. "Venezuelan Equine Encephalitis Virus Capsid Protein Inhibits Nuclear Import in Mammalian but Not in Mosquito Cells." *Journal of Virology* 82 (2008): 4028–4041.

Attoui, H., F. M. Jaafar, M. Belhouchet, et al. "*Micromonas pusilla* reovirus: A New Member of the Family *Reoviridae* Assigned to a Novel Proposed Genus (*Mimoreovirus*)." *Journal of General Virology* 87 (2006): 1375–1383.

Boonyaratanakornkit, J. B., E. J. Bartlett, E. Amaro-Carambot, and P. L. Collins. "The C Proteins of Human Parainfluenza Virus Type 1 (HPIV1) Control the Transcription of a Broad Array of Cellular Genes That Would Otherwise Respond to HPIV1 Infection." *Journal of Virology* 83 (2009): 1893–1910.

Braun D.K., Dominguez G., Pellett P.E. "Human herpesvirus 6." *Clinical Microbiology Reviews*, 10(1997): 521-567.

Chandran, K., D. L. Farsetta, and M. L. Nibert. "Strategy for Nonenveloped Virus Entry: A Hydrophobic Conformer of the Reovirus Membrane Penetration Protein μ1 Mediates Membrane Disruption." *Journal of Virology* 76 (2002): 9920–9933.

Chen, Y. B., A. Rahemtullah, and E. Hochberg. "Primary Effusion Lymphoma." *The Oncologist* 12 (2007): 569–576.

Cohen, J. Calling All Baby Boomers: Get Your Hepatitis C Test." *Science* 337 (2012): 903.

Cureton, D. K., R. H. Massol, S. Saffarian, T. L. Kirchhausen, and P. J. Whelan. "Vesicular Stomatitis Virus Enters Cells through Vesicles Incompletely Coated with Clathrin That Depend upon Actin for Internalization." *PLoS Pathogens* 5 (2009): e1000394.

Cuyck, H., J. Fan, D. L. Robertson, and P. Roques. "Evidence of Recombination between Divergent Hepatitis E Viruses." *Journal of Virology* 79 (2005): 9306–9314.

Dennehy, P. H. "Rotavirus Vaccines: An Overview." *Clinical Microbiology Reviews* 21 (2008):198–208.

Desforges, M., J. Desjardins, C. Zang, and P. J. Talbot. "The Acetyl-esterase Activity of the Hemagglutinin-esterase (HE) Protein of Human Coronavirus OC43 Strongly Enhances the Production of Infectious Virus." *Journal of Virology* (2013). doi: 10.1128/JVI.02699-12

Dong, C., J. Meng, X. Dai, J. H. Liang, et al. "Restricted Enzooticity of Hepatitis E Virus Genotypes 1 to 4 in the United States." *Journal of Clinical Microbiology* 49 (2011): 4164–4172.

Eggers, H. "Milestones in Early Poliomyelitis Research (1840 to 1949)." *Journal of Virology* 73 (1999): 4533–4535.

Engelkirk, P. G. and J. Duben-Engelkirk. *Laboratory Diagnosis of Infectious Diseases.* Baltimore, Maryland: Lippincott Williams and Wilkins, a Wolters Kluwer business, 2008: 734.

Emerson, S. U., H. Nguyen, U. Torian, and R. H. Purcell. "ORF3 Protein of Hepatitis E Virus Is Not Required for Replication, Virion Assembly, or Infection of Hepatoma Cells In Vitro." *Journal of Virology* 80 (2006): 10457–10464.

Farkas, T., K. Sestak, C. Wei, and X. Jiang. "Characterization of a Rhesus Monkey Calicivirus Representing a New Genus of *Caliciviridae.*" *Journal of Virology* 82 (2008): 5408–5416.

Fotedar, R., D. Stark, N. Beebe, D. Marriott, J. Ellis, and J. Harkness. "Laboratory Diagnostic Techniques for *Entamoeba* Species." *Clinical Microbiology Reviews* ASM 20 (2007): 511–532.

Gardner, C. L., C. W. Burke, M. Z. Tesfay, P. J. Glass, W. B. Klimstra, and K. D. Ryman. "Eastern and Venezuelan Equine Encephalitis Viruses Differ in Their Ability to Infect Dendritic Cells and Macrophages: Impact of Altered Cell Tropism on Pathogenesis." *Journal of Virology* 82 (2008): 10634–10646.

Halder, S., R. Ng, and M. Agbandje-McKenna. "Parvoviruses: Structure and Infection." *Future Virology* 7 (2012): 253–278.

Hall, C. B. "Respiratory Syncytial Virus and Parainfluenzae Virus." *New England Journal of Medicine* 344 (2001):1917–1928.

Henrickson, K. J. "Parainfluenza Viruses." *Clinical Microbiology Review* 16 (2003):242–264.

Hill, A. and Cooke G. Hepatitis C can be cured globally, but at what cost? *Science* 345 (2014): 141-142.

Huang, C. R. and S. J. Lo. "Evolution and Diversity of the Human Hepatitis D Virus Genome." *Advances in Bioinformatics.* 2010. doi:10.1155/2010/323654.

Johnson, B. W., O. Kosoy, E. Wang, M. Delorey, B. Russell, R. A. Bowen, and S. C. Weaver. "Use of Sindbis/Eastern

Equine Encephalitis Chimeric Viruses in Plaque Reduction Neutralization Tests for Arboviral Disease Diagnostics." *Clinical and Vaccine Immunology* 18 (2011):1486–1491.

Kaufmann, B., A. A. Simpson, and M. G. Rossmann. "The Structure of Human Parvovirus B19." *Proceedings of the National Academy of Sciences of the United States of America* 101 (2004): 11628–11633.

Kobiler, O., P. Brodersen, M. P. Taylor, E. B. Ludmir, and Enquist. "Herpesvirus Replication Compartments Originate with Single Incoming Viral Genomes." *mBio*, 2 (2011): e00278–11.

Kou, Z., M. Quinn, W. W. Rodrigo, R. C. Rose, *et al.* "Monocytes, but not T or B cells, Are the Principal Target Cells for Dengue Virus (DV) Infection among Human Peripheral Blood Mononuclear Cells." *Journal of Medical Virology* 80 (2008): 134–46.

Kramer, M. F., W. J. Cook, F. P. Roth, J. Zhu, H. Holman, D. M. Knipe, and D. M. Coen. "Latent Herpes Simplex Virus Infection of Sensory Neurons Alters Neuronal Gene Expression." *Journal of Virology* 77 (2003): 9533–9541.

Lambert, A. J., D. A. Martin, and R. S. Lanciotti. "Detection of North American Eastern and Western Equine Encephalitis Viruses by Nucleic Acid Amplification Assays." *Journal of Clinical Microbiology* 41 (2003): 379–385.

Lo, M. K., L. Lowe, Hummel, *et al.* "Characterization of Nipah Virus from Outbreaks in Bangladesh, 2008–2010." *Emerging Infectious Diseases* 18 (2012): 248–255.

Lu, B., R. Brazas, C. H. Ma, T. Kristoff, X. Cheng, and H. Jin. 2002. "Identification of Temperature-Sensitive Mutations in the Phosphoprotein of Respiratory Syncytial Virus That Are Likely Involved in Its Interaction with the Nucleoprotein." *Journal of Virology* 76 (2002): 2871–2880.

Mandel, E. D. "Erythema Infectiosum: Recognizing the Many Faces of Fifth Disease." *Journal of the American Academy of Physician Assistants* 22 (2002): 42–45.

Mahiet, C., A. Ergani, N. Huot, N. Alende, A. Azough, et al. Structural Variability of the Herpes Simplex Virus Type 1 Genome *in*

Vitro and *in Vivo.*" *Journal of Virology* (2012). doi:10.1128/JVI.00223-12.

Mani, A., S. M. Meraji, R. Houshyar, J. Radhakrishnan, A. Mani, M. Ahangar, T. M. Rezaie, M. A. Taghavinejad, B. Broumand, H. Zhao, C. Nelson-Williams, and R. P. Lifton. "Finding Genetic Contributions to Sporadic Disease: A Recessive Locus at 12q24 Commonly Contributes to Patent Ductus Arteriosus." *Proceedings of Natural Academy of Sciences of the United States of America* 99 (2002): 15054–15059.

Matsuura, M., M. Takemoto, K. Yamanishi, and Y. Mori. "Human Herpesvirus 6 Major Immediate Early Promoter Has Strong Activity in T Cells and Is Useful for Heterologous Gene Expression." *Virology Journal* 8 (2011): 9.

Merens, A., P. J. Guerin, J. P. Guthmann, and E. Nicand. "Outbreak of Hepatitis E Virus Infection in Darfur, Sudan: Effectiveness of Real-Time Reverse Transcription-PCR Analysis of Dried Blood Spots." *Journal of Clinical Microbiology* 47 (2009): 1931–1933.

Miyazaki, N., T. Uehara-Ichiki, L. Xing, L. Bergman, et al. "Structural Evolution of *Reoviridae* Revealed by *Oryzavirus* in Acquiring the Second Capsid Shell." *Journal of Virology* 82 (2008): 11344–11353.

Mohamadzadeh, M., S. S. Coberley, G. G. Olinger, W. V. Kalina, G. Ruthel, et al. "Activation of Triggering Receptor Expressed on Myeloid Cells-1 on Human Neutrophils by Marburg and Ebola Viruses." *Journal of Virology* 80 (2006): 7235–7244.

Mohr S., S. Grandemange, P. Massimi, G. Darai, L. Banks, J. C. Martinou, M. Zeier, and W. Muranyi. "Targeting the Retinoblastoma Protein by MC007L, Gene Product of the Molluscum Contagiosum Virus: Detection of a Novel Virus-Cell Interaction by a Member of the Poxviruses." *Journal of Virology* 82 (2008): 10625–10633.

Moscona, A. "Entry of Parainfluenza Virus into Cells as a Target for Interrupting Childhood Respiratory Disease." *The Journal of Clinical Investigation* 115 (2005): 1688–1698.

Murray, K., C. Walker, E. Herrington, J. A. Lewis, J. McCormick, D. W. C. Beasley, R. B. Tesh, and S. Fisher-Hoch. "Persistent Infection with West Nile Virus Years after Initial Infection." *The Journal of Infectious Diseases* 1 (2010): 2–4.

Nishio, M., M. Tsurudome, M. Ito, M. Kawano, S. Kusagawa, H. Komada, and Y. Ito. "Mapping of Domains on the Human Parainfluenza Virus Type 2 Nucleocapsid Protein (NP) Required for NP–Phosphoprotein or NP–NP Interaction." *Journal of General Virology* 80 (1999): 2017–2022.

Palmer, S. G., M. Porotto, L. M. Palermo, L. Cinha, O. Creengard, and A. Moscona. "Adaptation of Human Parainfluenza Virus to Airway Epithelium Reveals Fusion Properties Required for Growth in Host Tissue." *mBio* 3 (2012): e00137-12.

Parrish, C. R. "Structures and Functions of Parvovirus Capsids and the Process of Cell Infection." *Current Topics in Microbiology and Immunology* 343 (2010): 149–76.

Petrakova, O., E. Volkova, R. Gorchakov, S. Paessler, R. M. Kinney, and I. Frolov. "Noncytopathic Replication of Venezuelan Equine Encephalitis Virus and Eastern Equine Encephalitis Virus Replicons in Mammalian Cells." *Journal of Virology* 79 (2005): 7597–7608.

Pica, F. and A. Volpi. "Transmission of Human Herpesvirus 8: An Update." *Current Opinion in Infectious Diseases* 20 (2007): 152–6.

Ohkawa, T., L. E. Volkman, and M. Welch. "Actin-Based Motility Drives Baculovirus Transit to the Nucleus and Cell Surface." *The Journal of Experimental Medicine* 190 (2010): 187–195.

O'Keefe, B. R., B. Giomarelli, D. L. Barnard, S. R. Shenoy, P. K. S. Chan, et al. "Broad-Spectrum *In Vitro* Activity and *In Vivo* Efficacy of the Antiviral Protein Griffithsin against Emerging Viruses of the Family *Coronaviridae*." *Journal of Virology* 84 (2010): 2511–2521.

Ouzilou, L., E. Caliot, I. Pelletier, et al. "Poliovirus Transcytosis through M-Like Cells." *Journal of General Virology* 83 (2002): 2177–2182.

Overby, A. K., V. Popov, E. P. A. Neve, and R. F. Pettersson. "Generation and Analysis of Infectious Virus-Like Particles of Uukuniemi Virus (*Bunyaviridae*): A Useful System for Studying Bunyaviral Packaging and Budding." *Journal of Virology* 80 (2006): 10428–10435.

Roberts, L. "Fighting Polio in Pakistan." *Science* 337 (2012): 517–521.

Roberts, L. "The Polio Emergency." *Science* 337 (2012): 497–612.

Schultz, M. "Theobald Smith." *Emerging Infectious Diseases* 14 (2008): 1940–1942.

Selariu, A., T. Cheng, Q. Tang, B. Silver, L. Yang, C. Liu, et al. "ORF7 of Varicella Zoster Virus is a Neurotropic Factor." *Journal of Virology* (2012). doi: 10.1128/JVI.00128-12

Sherman, I. W. *Twelve Diseases that Changed Our World*. Washington, DC: ASM Press, 2007. 219.

Sherman, M. B. and S. C. Weaver. "Structure of the Recombinant Alphavirus Western Equine Encephalitis Virus Revealed by Cryoelectron Microscopy." *Journal of Virology* 84 (2010): 9775–9782.

Sillender, W. M. "Respiratory Syncytial Virus Genetic and Antigenic Diversity." *Clinical Microbiology Review* 13 (2000): 1–15.

Simpson, A. A., B. HeAbert, G. M. Sullivan, C. R. Parrish, Z. ZaAdori, P. Tijssen, and M. G. Rossmann. "The Structure of Porcine Parvovirus: Comparison with Related Viruses." *Journal of Molecular Biology* 315 (2002): 1189–1198.

Steele, K. E., A. O. Anderson, and M. Mohamadzadeh. "Fibroblastic Reticular Cells and Their Role in Viral Hemorrhagic Fevers." *Expert Review of Anti-Infective Therapy* 7 (2009): 423–435.

Strokes, K., M. H. Chi, K. Sakamoto, D. C. Newcomb, M. G. Currier. "Differential Pathogenesis of Respiratory Syncytial Virus Clinical Isolates in BALB/c Mice." *Journal of Virology* 85 (2011): 5782–5793.

Tsai, B. "Penetration of nonenveloped viruses into the cytoplasm." *Annual Review of Cell and Developmental Biology* 23 (2007): 23–43.

Tuddenham, L., J. S. Jung, B. Chane-Woon-Ming, L. Dolken, and S. Pfeffer. "Small RNA Deep Sequencing Identifies MicroRNAs and Other Small Noncoding RNAs from Human Herpesvirus 6B." *Journal of Virology* 86 (2011): 1638–1649.

Tuffereau, C., K. Schmidt, C. Langevin, F. Lafay, G. Dechant, and M. Koltzenburg. "The Rabies Virus Glycoprotein Receptor p75[NTR] Is Not Essential for Rabies Virus Infection." *Journal of Virology*, 81 (2007):13622–13630.

UNAIDS World AIDS Day Report. 2011.

Van de Perre, P., P. A. Rubbo, J. Viljoen, N. Nagot, T. Tylleskar, et al. "HIV-1 Reservoirs in Breast Milk and Challenges to Elimination of Breast-Feeding Transmission of HIV-1." *Science Translational Medicine* 4 (2012):143.

Vihinen-Ranta, M., S. Suikkanen, and C. R. Parrish. "Pathways of Cell Infection by Parvoviruses and Adeno-Associated Viruses." *Journal of Virology* 78 (2004): 6709–6714.

Wang, L., L. Longding, Y. Che, L. Wang, L. Jiang, et al. "Egress of HSV-1 Capsid Requires the Interaction of VP26 and a Cellular Tetraspanin Membrane Protein." *Virology Journal* 7 (2010): 156.

Weli, S. C., C. A. Scott, C. A. Ward, and A. C. Jackson. "Rabies Virus Infection of Primary Neuronal Cultures and Adult Mice: Failure to Demonstrate Evidence of Excitotoxicity." *Journal of Virology* 80 (2006): 10270–10273.

World Health Organization. World Malaria Report, 2010.

Xiang, Y. and B. Moss. "Molluscum Contagiosum Virus Interleukin-18 (IL-18) Binding Protein Is Secreted as a Full-Length Form That Binds Cell Surface Glycosaminoglycans through the C-Terminal Tail and a Furin-Cleaved Form with Only the IL-18 Binding Domain." *Journal of Virology* 77 (2003): 2623–2630.

Zhang, M., Y. Fang, A. C. Brault, and W. K. Reisen. "Variation in Western Equine Encephalomyelitis Viral Strain Growth in Mammalian, Avian, and Mosquito Cells Fails to Explain Temporal Changes in Enzootic and Epidemic Activity in California." *Vector-Borne and Zoonotic Diseases* 11 (2011): 269–275.

INDEX

W

Y

Z